SLIMMING

One Pound Meals

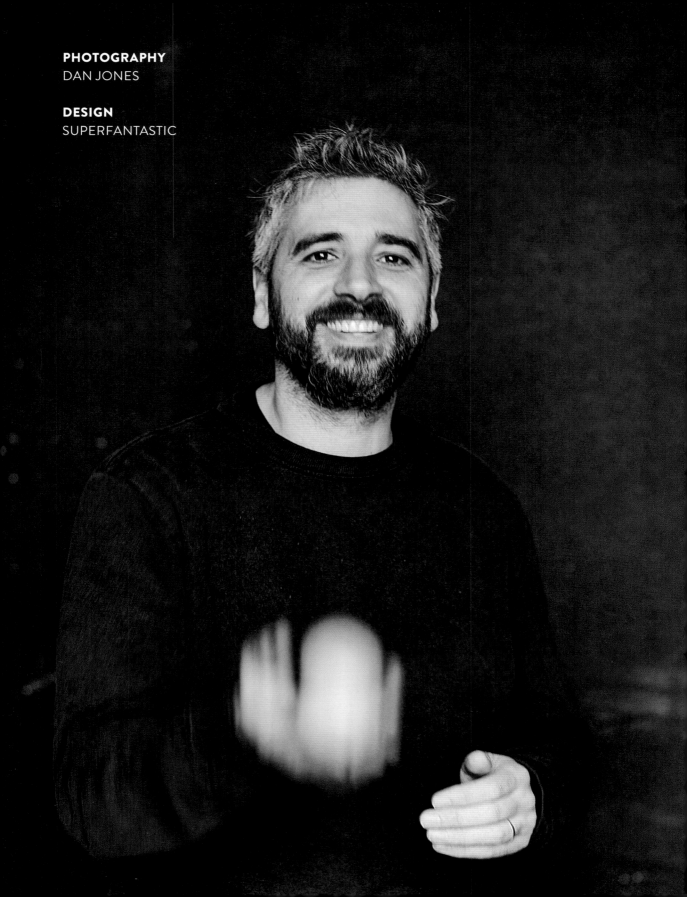

PHOTOGRAPHY
DAN JONES

DESIGN
SUPERFANTASTIC

SLIMMING

One Pound Meals

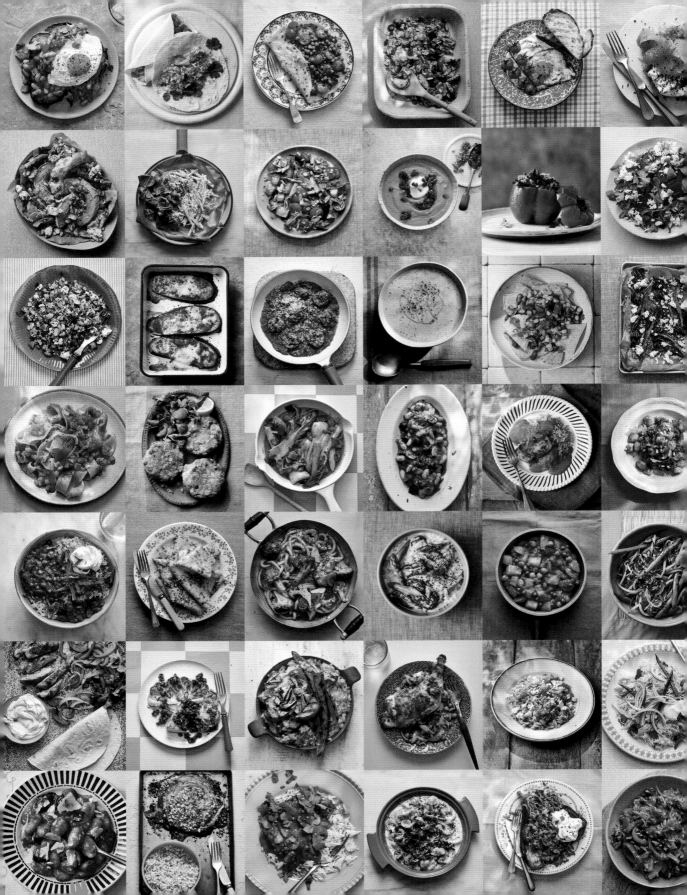

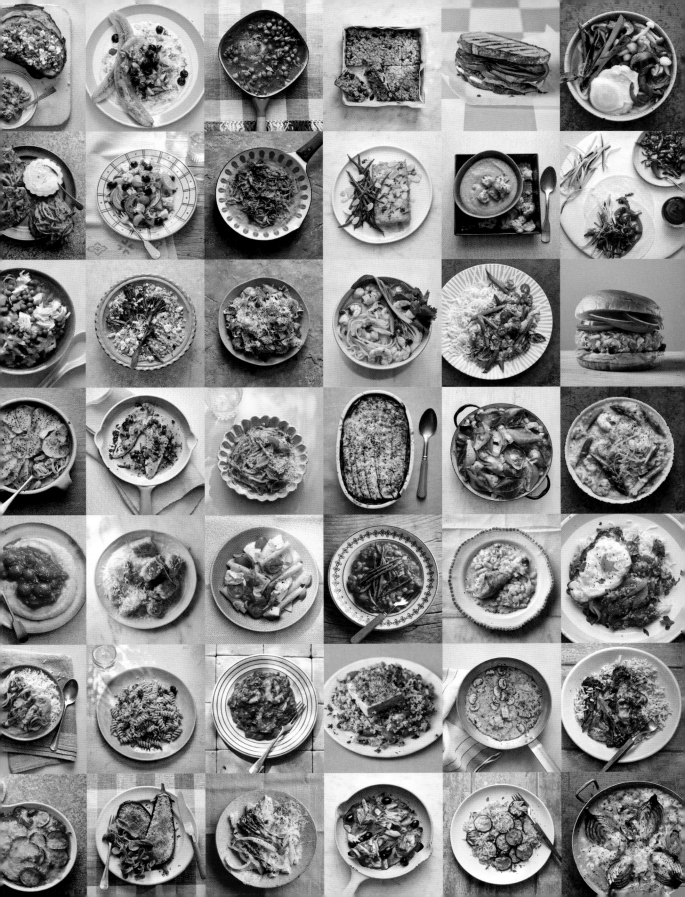

CONTENTS

DINNER

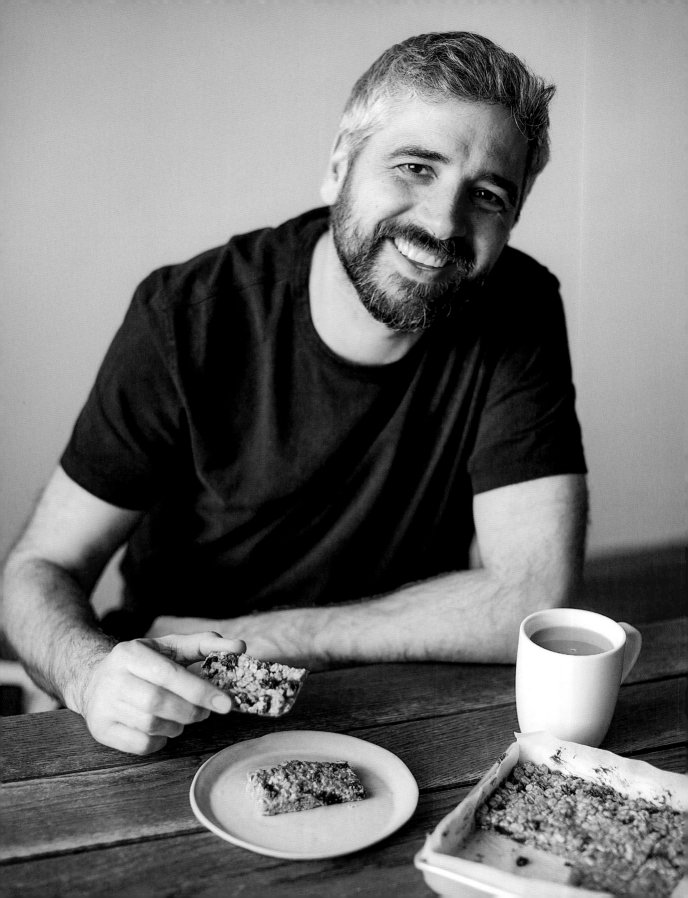

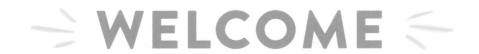

WELCOME

I'm back! My latest book in the One Pound Meals series is all about healthier meals that can help with weight loss. I know it can be a bit daunting changing your long-term habits, so what I've done is just slightly tweak my usual thing to make it an easy and realistic transition for you. I'm still using the same ingredients, and still cooking in my no-frills style with the usual hacks that make it all so effortless.

WHAT ARE £1 MEALS?

As the name suggests, these are all meals that cost £1 to make. And just like with all my previous books, I've simplified and slimmed down (pun intended!) the number of ingredients in order to hit that £1 target – so they're all super simple. These are the characteristics of my cooking, and this approach is what makes my recipes so accessible. They are easy because they use ingredients you are already familiar with. This is certainly not classical cooking using traditional techniques; this is cooking you can actually do after a day's work, cooking that can slip easily into your daily routine without much hassle.

WHY HAVE I WRITTEN A SLIMMING BOOK?

This isn't a book about my 'slimming journey'. But a while back, I did some work with Lorraine Kelly for a weight-loss company, and found that my style of cooking effortlessly transitioned into weight-loss recipes. I started getting interested in exactly what I was eating. I started swapping a few things here and there. There was no big change or overhaul, but after making these swaps, I felt I had more energy and I was in better shape.

I've never mentioned this in my books before, but quite randomly, I actually have a degree in biochemistry, so I have a better-than-average grasp of the human body and understand things at a molecular level. I used to read scientific papers and wear a white lab coat and safety specs. This means I can cut through the hype, and I'm not easily convinced of anything that is not proper science. There are so many weight-loss diets out there that it can be confusing, but it doesn't have to be. The most popular weight-loss concepts are calorie control/fasting and reducing carbohydrates. So, I've created 86 recipes that can fit in with either of these approaches. This book can work for you whether you're on a low-carb, low-calorie or fasting diet.

I think I might have found the most hassle-free and sustainable way to help you keep on top of your weight!

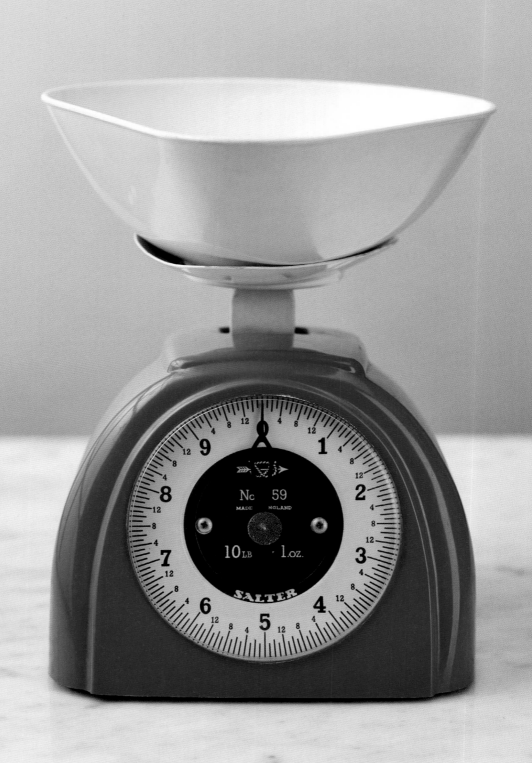

WHAT IS A LOW-CALORIE DIET?

The weight-loss approach that has, without doubt, been the most popular over the last century is that of counting calories. And I agree that it can be a helpful strategy. With a few small changes and an understanding of what goes into the food you eat, you can cut some needless calories out of your diet and still enjoy satisfying meals. It makes scientific sense, and by not doing anything too drastic, there's a far greater chance it will become a long-term habit that you actually manage to stick to.

WHAT IS FASTING?

A few fasting diets have become popular recently. I've looked at the science, I understand the concept, and yes, it makes sense from a scientific standpoint. All the recipes in this book are under 500 calories, and so can fit in with your fasting programme, whether you're sticking to a certain number of calories a day or fasting for a couple of days a week. Many of the recipes are well under 500 calories, such as the Aubergine Pizzette (page 76), which contains 112 calories per portion, and the Cauliflower Chop with Caper Salsa Verde (page 152), which contains only 74 calories!

WHAT IS A LOW-CARBOHYDRATE DIET?

In recent years, the popularity of the low-carb diet has made a huge impact, so I have included some nice options for this, too. You don't have to jump through many hoops to prepare a low-carb meal, and they are still fun, exciting and delicious recipes that you will look forward to eating. Low-carb diets have been shown to be helpful for weight loss and health in general, so check out the Halloumi Chopped Salad (page 52), which has only 11.7g carbohydrates or the Flattened Chicken with Caper Jus (page 116), with 0.3g. One of the effects of a low-carb diet is that it can help keep your blood sugar balanced, which helps with burning fat. How much carbohydrate should you be eating a day? It depends on you and your goals, but 50–100g is generally considered low carb.

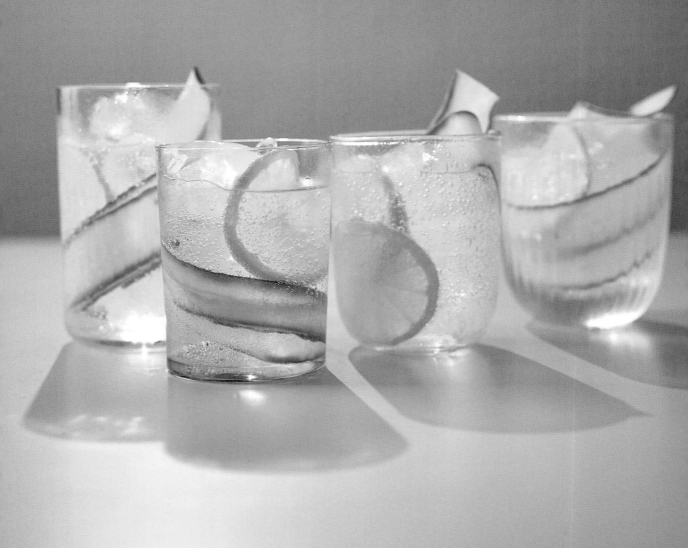

BLOOD-SUGAR BALANCE AND WHY IT'S SO IMPORTANT

Keeping your blood sugar balanced is one of the most important things you can do for your health. Blood-sugar balance affects everything from energy levels and weight to sleep and mood. Long-term blood-sugar imbalance can lead to insulin resistance, which is a risk factor for diabetes, dementia and heart disease. So, keeping blood-sugar levels balanced is super important.

How do we do it? Firstly, by eating balanced meals with protein, fat and complex carbs.

When it comes to carbs, it's all about the right kind. Carbohydrates have the greatest effect on our blood-sugar levels. We want to reduce simple carbs – sugar – and instead choose complex carbs, such as vegetables, grains and legumes, which contain the all-important fibre. We also don't want to eat too many carbs in general, and you might even choose to follow a low-carb diet.

Protein is really important for lots of things in the body, but one of its benefits is that it can help keep blood-sugar levels stable, and it also keeps you full for longer. Making sure your meals have a good protein source can be effective for weight loss.

Fats hardly affect blood sugar, and they're also really filling, so they can prevent us from eating too much. We need to choose the right kinds of fat, though, and avoid high-fat processed foods.

EXERCISE

The final concept I want to talk about is exercise. I know exercise is essential for living a long and healthy life, but I just find it so difficult to actually schedule any exercise into my weekly routine. My way around this is to just lead a more active life every day. By walking instead of catching the bus, or doing some DIY, I stay pretty active but without the pressure of having to schedule it into my routine. This is all part of my philosophy of making it easy for myself and just making a few tweaks here and there so it's not a daunting uphill struggle.

Oh, I almost forgot – drink loads of water too. It's an easy one to get you on the right track, doesn't take much effort and it counts as a win for the day.

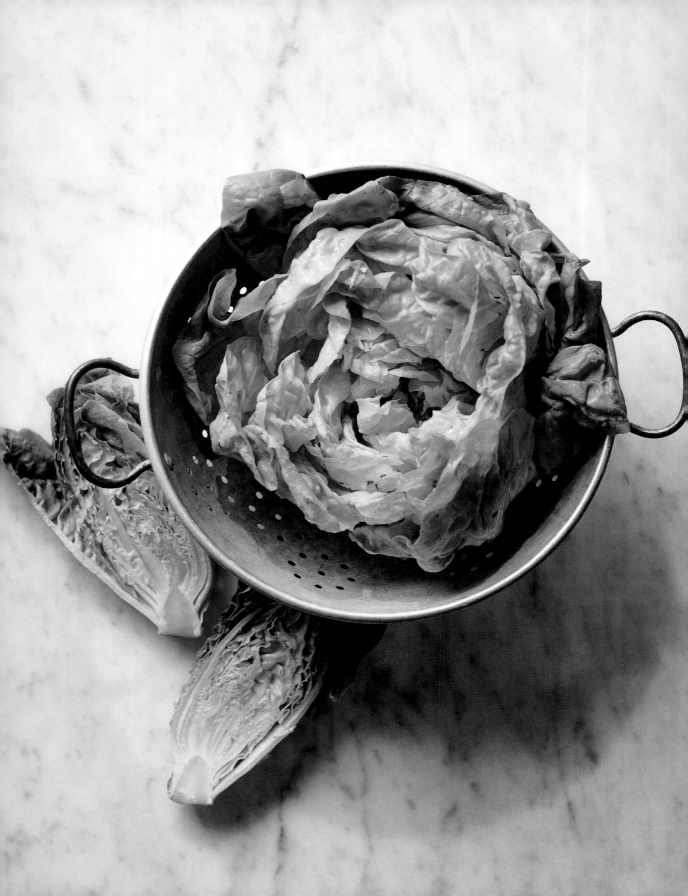

HANDY SWAPS

Making swaps is one of the key things you can do to transform your diet and your health. Just gradually swap your usual choices for healthier versions, and soon enough it will become second nature to you.

- Wholegrain versions of staples such as pasta and bread are just as tasty, and are normally right there on the supermarket shelf next to your usual choice. They contain more fibre, so are better for balancing your blood sugar.

- Courgette slices are a brilliant low-carb alternative to lasagne sheets.

- Lower-carb vegetables, such as butternut squash and cauliflower, are a great substitute for potatoes.

- Bulk up your meals with vegetables – for example, substitute half the pasta in a dish with broccoli (see my Quick Broccoli & Chilli Pasta on page 164).

- Eat lots of veg in general – vegetables like broccoli, cauliflower, courgettes and aubergine contain lots of fibre, so are great for blood-sugar balance. They are also full of vitamins and minerals, so they can make you feel great too.

- Eggs are a great low-carb option for breakfast. Avoid sugary breakfast cereals.

- Lentils and beans are so cheap, and they're full of protein and fibre to keep you full for longer.

- Soups are a brilliant slimming hack. They're really filling, cheap, and a great way to use up any leftover bits in your fridge or store cupboard.

LOW-CALORIE HACKS

- Replace meat with veg, like in my Aubergine 'Bacon' BLT (see page 44).

- Cooking fats and oils contain a lot of calories, so be careful that you only use a small amount. All my recipes say to use a splash of oil, which is about a teaspoon.

- Minor adjustments, like using low-fat natural yoghurt instead of full fat or avoiding cream and other high-calorie ingredients when they're not needed can make a big difference (see my No-Cream Stroganoff recipe on page 172).

- Baking is a great alternative to deep-frying, which uses lots of oil (see my Oven Bhajis on page 60).

- Portion control is important for weight loss and using a smaller plate is a great hack for this. Simple but effective!

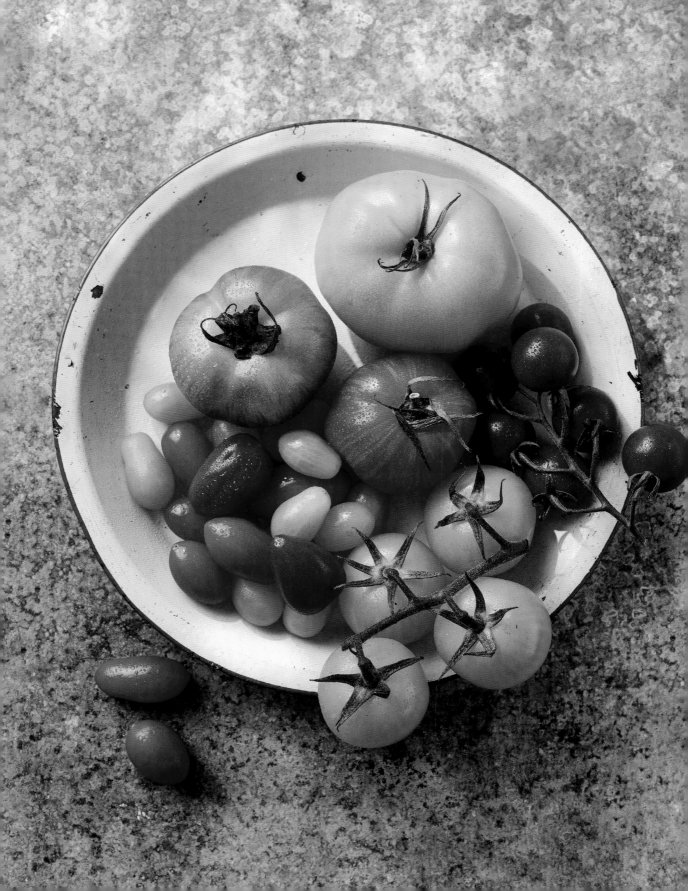

HOME COOKING VS TAKEAWAYS AND READY MEALS

For me, the most important thing when it comes to staying healthy is cooking my own food from scratch. Staying away from processed food, ready meals and takeaway foods that are laden with fats and sugars is key. The health benefits of cooking from scratch at home and seeing with your own eyes what is actually going into your meal will unlock a world of health and happiness.

And I would say this concept is probably the most important part of this book. How do you stay away from takeaways? Primarily by accepting that there are limitations on your time and ability to cook food at home. You need to be realistic about what is achievable when you get home from work. And that's where my lazy style of cooking with minimal ingredients comes in. This is the bare minimum required to get a tasty, inexpensive and healthy plate of food on the table. I'm not asking you to soak chickpeas overnight, brew stocks by boiling bones or make pastry from scratch. Why? Because even I can't be bothered to do that, and I'm a chef. This is modern home cooking, using modern conveniences that I have tailored to the modern pace of life.

HOW TO USE THIS BOOK

At the top of each recipe, you will be told how many calories and grams of carbohydrates it contains, and at the back of the book I've provided a table with more nutritional info. If you are following a specific diet, you can easily find the information you need.

I've also added **vegetarian**, **vegan**, **dairy-free** and **gluten-free** symbols to make it even easier to see which recipes are for you.

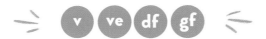

Of course, you can still use any of the recipes you like, even if you're not following a specific diet!

Do remember to check the label on things like stock cubes, which aren't always gluten-free.

This book is intended to fit in with your chosen diet plan. Not all diets are suitable for everyone. If you have any concerns, or if you have been prescribed a particular diet by your doctor or other healthcare professional, we recommend that you consult with your doctor before making any changes to your diet.

The nutritional figures given for each recipe are intended as a guide. The exact figures will depend on the specific ingredients used and portion size.

The author and publisher disclaim any liability incurred directly or indirectly from the use of the material in this book by any person.

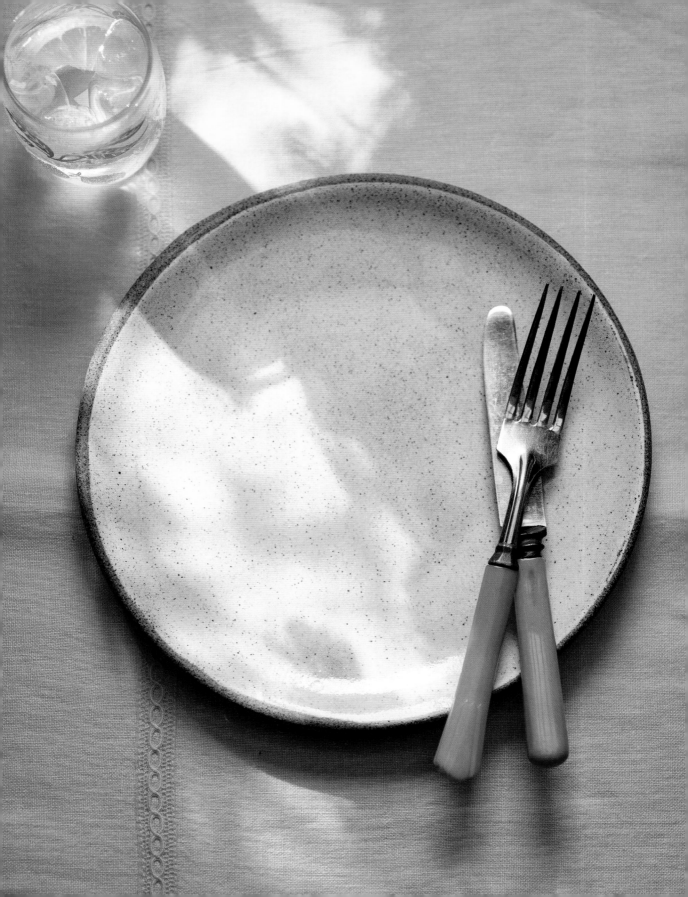

ALL RECIPES
ARE FOR A SINGLE SERVING

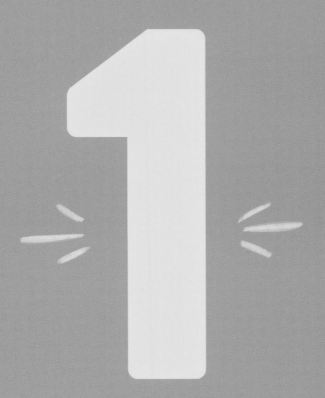

MORE THAN ONE PERSON?
Just adjust to suit your circumstances.

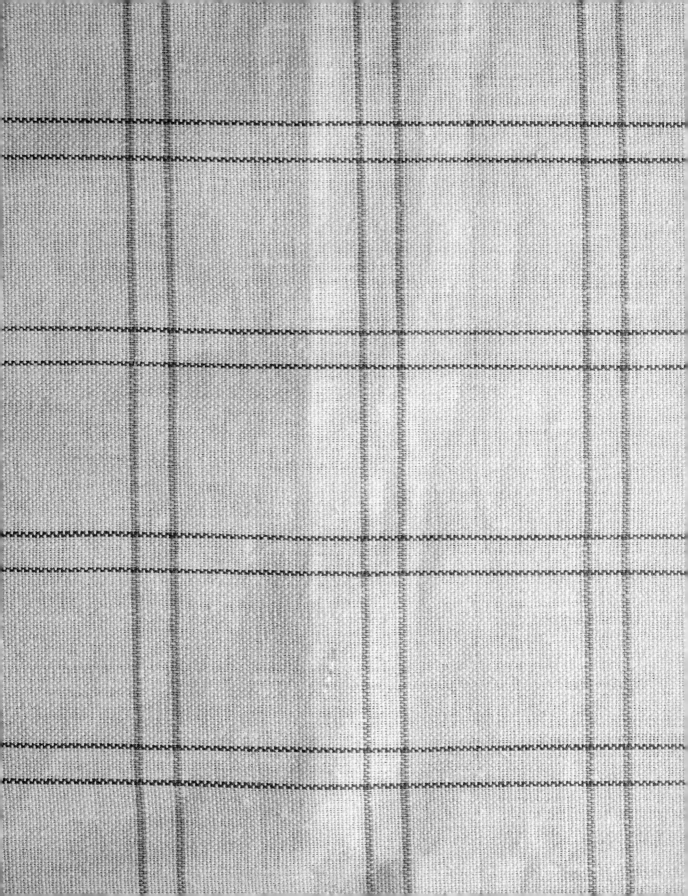

BREAKFAST & BRUNCH

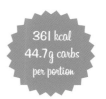

361 kcal
44.7g carbs
per portion

SMOKY BEANS ON TOAST

The perfect brunch recipe, packed with protein-rich beans. Best of all, it contains zero added sugar. By making your own homemade versions of things like baked beans, you know exactly what's in the food you're eating.

To make 1 portion

¼ red pepper, seeded and sliced

¼ tin of cannellini beans (100g)

¼ tin of chopped tomatoes (100g)

Pinch of smoked paprika

Splash of Worcestershire sauce (optional)

2 slices of bread

1 egg

Small handful of chopped coriander

Oil (any)

Salt and pepper

To cook

Pan-fry the red pepper in a splash of oil over a medium heat for a few minutes before adding the beans and the chopped tomatoes. Season with salt, pepper, paprika and a splash of Worcestershire sauce (if using), then simmer for about 10 minutes (adding a splash of water if it gets too dry).

Meanwhile, toast the bread (either in a toaster or in a griddle pan, if you want those char marks), and fry the egg.

Assemble your breakfast, garnish with coriander and serve.

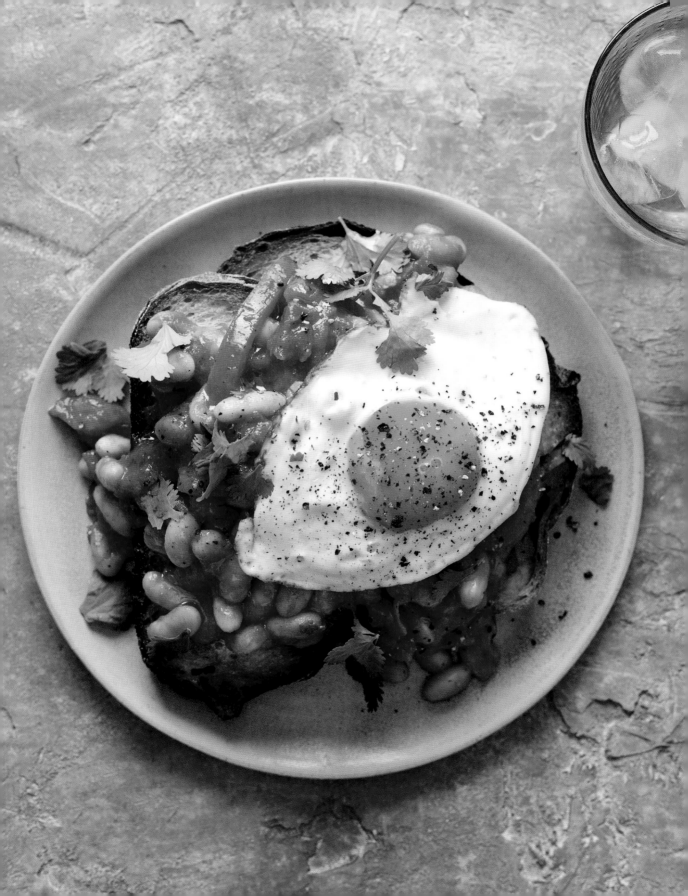

BREAKFAST EGG TACOS

Jazzing up your scrambled egg with onions, peppers and paprika, and then wrapping it all up in a tortilla is a great way to start the day. You don't need much onion or pepper, so I've measured them in tablespoons. This might seem strange, but the idea is to keep a little aside from a main meal from earlier in the week.

To make 1 portion (2 tacos)

1 tbsp diced red onion

1 tbsp diced red pepper

1 egg

2 small tortilla wraps

Pinch of paprika

Small handful of chopped coriander

Oil (any)

Salt and pepper

To cook

Pan-fry the onion and red pepper in a splash of oil over a medium–high heat for a couple of minutes to soften, then crack in the egg, season and mix it all together to scramble the egg. Cook for another couple of minutes, then spoon the scrambled egg on to the tortillas and top with a little pinch of paprika and a sprinkle of chopped coriander. Roll up and serve.

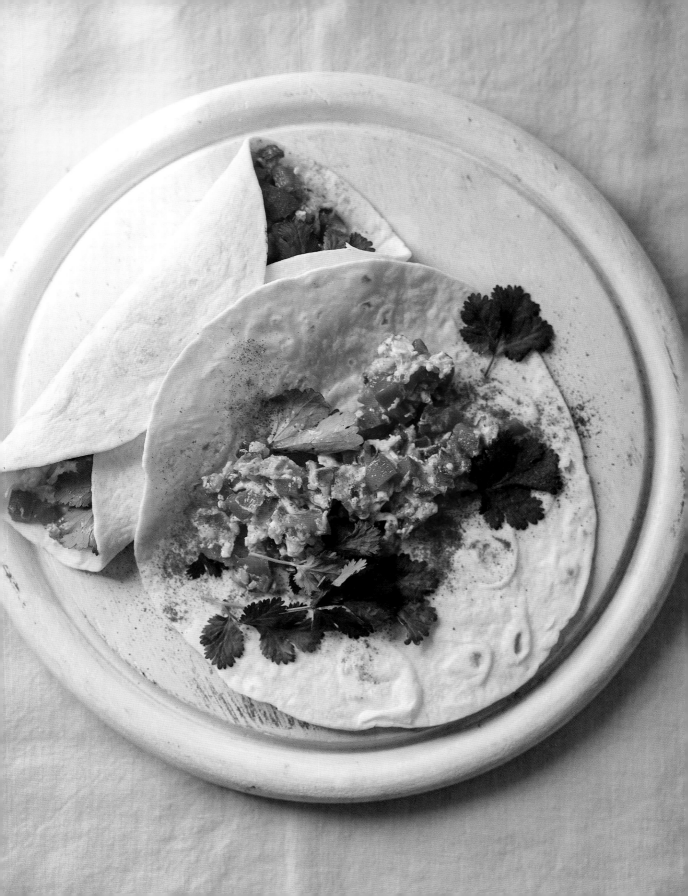

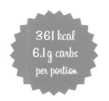

361 kcal
6.1g carbs
per portion

TOMATO & BACON BREAKFAST OMELETTE

A filling way to start the day. I've taken some of the flavours of a full English, but adapted them to make this tasty breakfast option. And for a bit of colour and some added nutrients, I've chucked in a few peas, too.

To make 1 portion

2 rashers bacon

A few cherry tomatoes, halved

Small handful of frozen peas

3 eggs

Sprinkle of chopped chives

Oil (any)

Salt and pepper

To cook

Pan-fry the bacon and tomatoes in a splash of oil over a medium heat for a few minutes on each side until the bacon is cooked.

Defrost the peas under the hot tap.

In a bowl, beat the eggs, then season and pour into a small, oiled frying pan. Cook over a medium heat for a couple of minutes until it's about half-cooked. Add the bacon, tomatoes and peas, then fold over the omelette. Cook for a couple more minutes until the egg mixture is set, then garnish with chopped chives and serve.

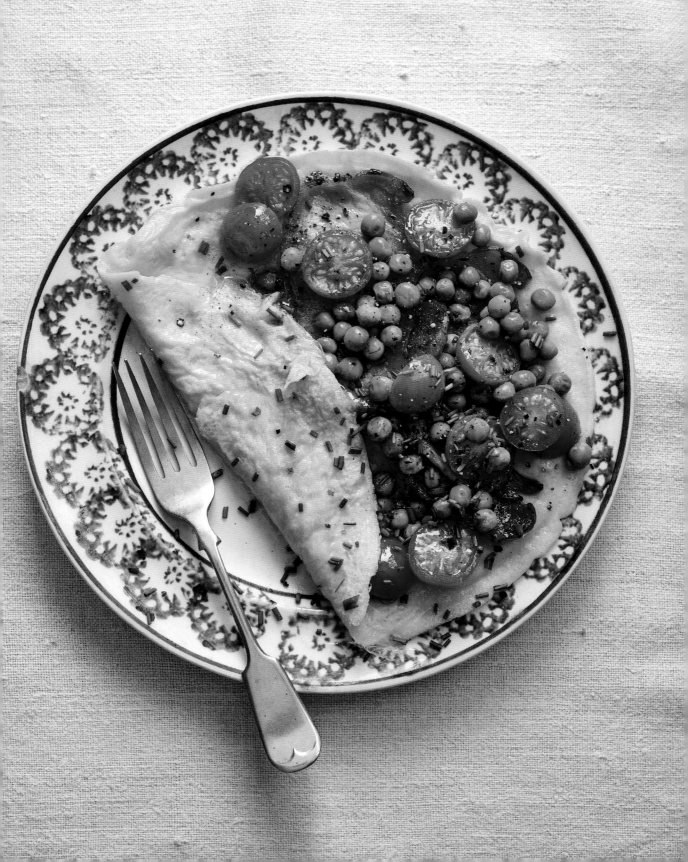

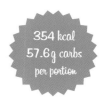

354 kcal
57.6g carbs
per portion

HONEY NUT & CRANBERRY GRANOLA

The problem with shop-bought cereals is that they are often loaded with refined sugars, salt and preservatives. So why not have a go at making some yourself? I like to make a huge batch of this granola and store it in a glass jar on the shelf because it looks so pretty. It's delicious served with milk or yoghurt.

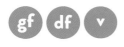

To make 1 portion

Handful of rolled oats

Handful of nuts (any)

Handful of dried cranberries (or any dried fruit)

1 tbsp honey

To cook

Preheat your oven to 180°C/gas mark 4 and line a baking sheet with baking parchment.

Mix together your oats, nuts and cranberries on the lined baking sheet, then drizzle with the honey. Mix again using a spoon and make sure the mixture is spread out evenly. Bake in the oven for 10 minutes, then leave to cool. Once cooled, break it up and serve.

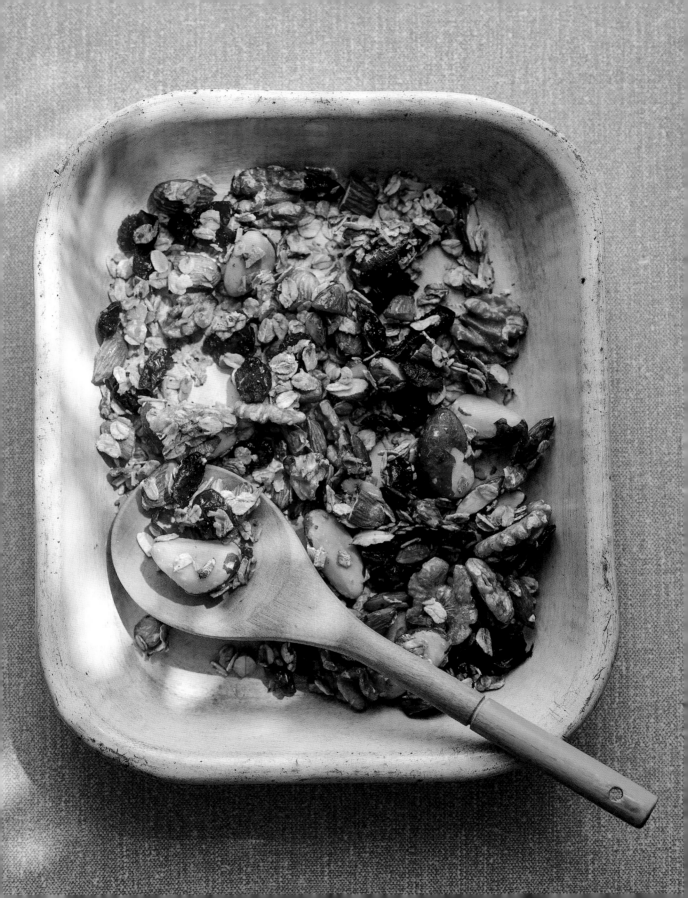

487 kcal
35.5 g carbs
per portion

SAVOURY BREAKFAST YOGHURT

This is a totally different approach to yoghurt! Beautifully roasted tomatoes, eggs and yoghurt . . . a great way to start the day. The roasted tomato juices bring it all together, so definitely spoon those over the top.

To make 1 portion

Handful of cherry vine tomatoes

Pinch of dried oregano

1 egg

4 tbsp Greek-style yoghurt

Slice of sourdough bread (optional)

Olive oil

Salt and pepper

To cook

Preheat your oven to 180°C/gas mark 4.

Chuck the tomatoes into a roasting tin, along with a glug of oil, the oregano and a pinch of salt and pepper. Roast for about 15 minutes until the tomatoes are soft and the juices have spilled out.

Meanwhile, either fry or poach the egg.

Spoon the yoghurt into a shallow bowl and top with the egg and tomatoes, then pour over the juices from the roasting tin. Serve with a slice of sourdough, if using.

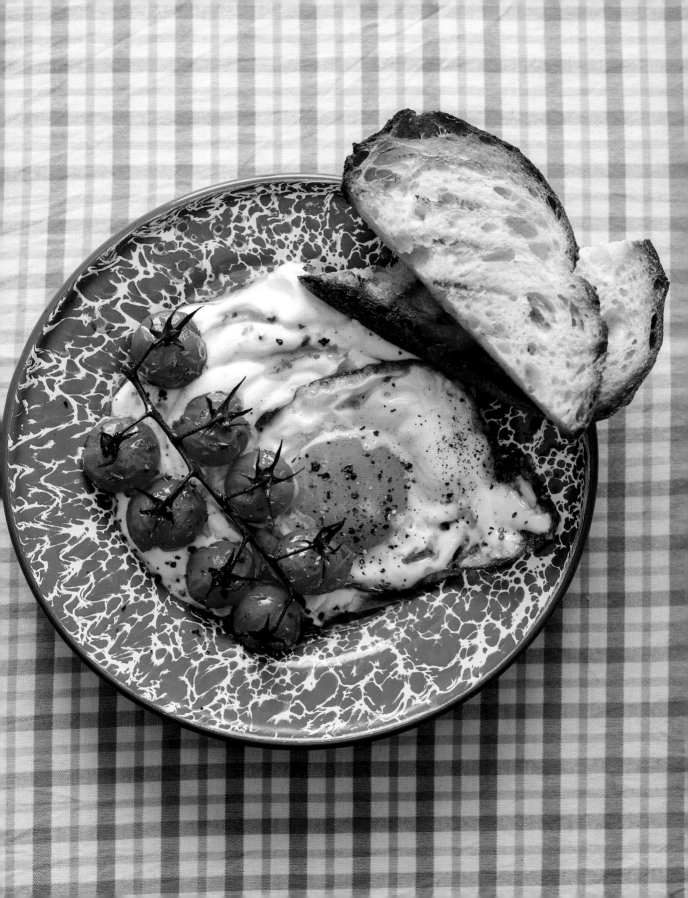

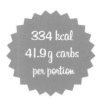

334 kcal
41.9g carbs
per portion

SMOKED SALMON ROSTI HACK

To make a rosti, normally you would grate a potato into a colander, lightly salt it, let it rest, then transfer it to a tea towel and wring it out to extract the water – and basically make as much mess as you possibly can. This is a huge obstacle that I just find too difficult first thing in the morning. So, I created a lazy way to do it. Just grate the potato directly into the pan and let the water evaporate off with the heat.

To make 1 portion

½ potato

½ tsp plain flour

Dollop of cream cheese

Slice of smoked salmon

Sprinkle of chopped chives

Oil (any)

Salt and pepper

To cook

Grate the potato directly into a lightly oiled pan over a medium heat. Season, add the flour and fry for about 5 minutes while moving it around with a wooden spoon so the water from the potato evaporates. Then form a rosti in the middle of the pan with a spoon and leave it for a few minutes while the shape sets. Flip it over and cook for a few more minutes on the other side. Once cooked and golden, transfer to a plate and top with a dollop of cream cheese and a slice of salmon. Sprinkle over some chopped chives, if using, and serve.

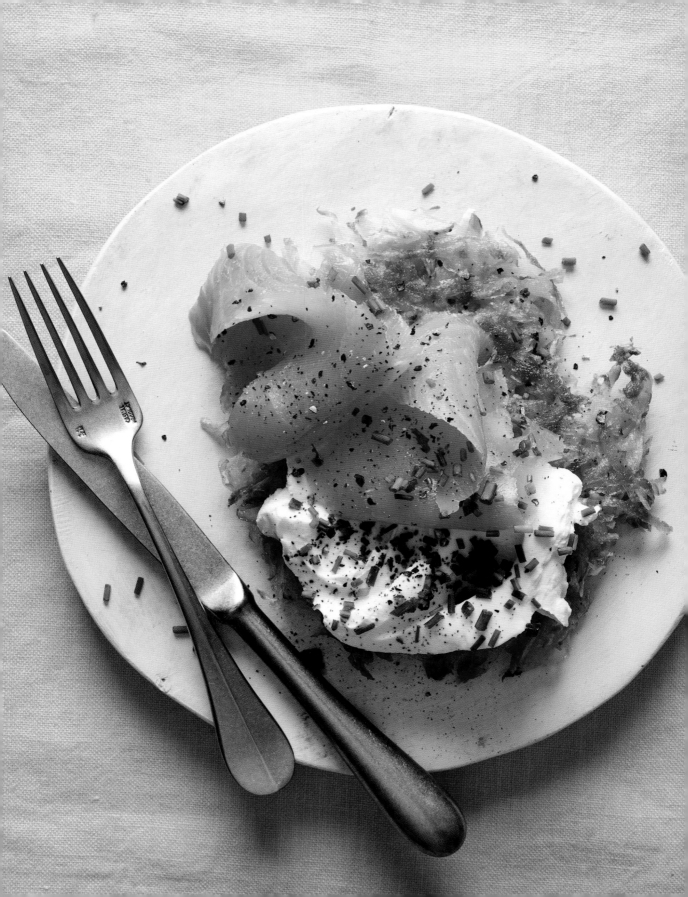

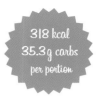
318 kcal
35.3g carbs
per portion

SMASHED PEA, AVOCADO & FETA

Avocado is expensive, so I've added peas to bulk it out. And why not? They're both green; they're both tasty. To elevate this dish from breakfast to brunch, I've added a bit of feta, with its lovely salty, tangy flavour. It's the perfect topping for your toast.

To make 1 portion

Small handful of frozen peas

¼ avocado

Pinch of dried chilli flakes

2 slices of bread

Small handful of crumbled feta

Olive oil

Salt and pepper

To cook

Defrost the peas under the hot tap, then tip into a bowl and add the avocado and a pinch of salt, pepper and chilli flakes, then mash with a fork.

Meanwhile, toast the bread, or, if you're feeling extra decadent, drizzle the bread with olive oil and sprinkle with salt, then griddle to get those char marks.

Dollop the avocado mixture on to the toast and top with the crumbled feta.

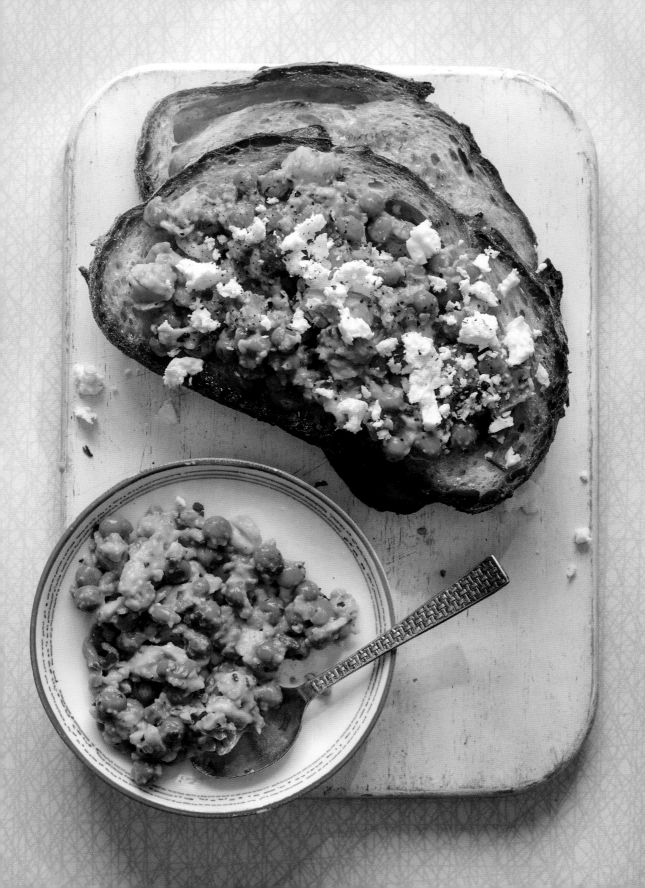

OVERNIGHT OATS

420 kcal
65.2 g carbs
per portion

Joe Wicks is often eating overnight oats for breakfast, and he looks great. I like to add a pinch of cinnamon to mine to make them taste a bit like rice pudding. It could be this addition of cinnamon that is keeping me from looking like Joe Wicks, but this recipe is definitely a step in the right direction.

To make 1 portion

¼ mug of rolled oats

¼ mug of milk

Pinch of ground cinnamon

1 banana

1 tsp honey

Small handful of crushed unsalted nuts (any kind)

A few blueberries

Oil (any)

To cook

The night before, tip the oats into a container with a lid, pour over the milk and add a pinch of cinnamon. Mix and cover with the lid, then refrigerate overnight.

In the morning, transfer the oats to a bowl and slice the banana in half lengthways. Pan-fry in a splash of oil over a medium–high heat for a few minutes until nicely caramelised, then add to the oats, along with a drizzle of honey, some crushed nuts and blueberries.

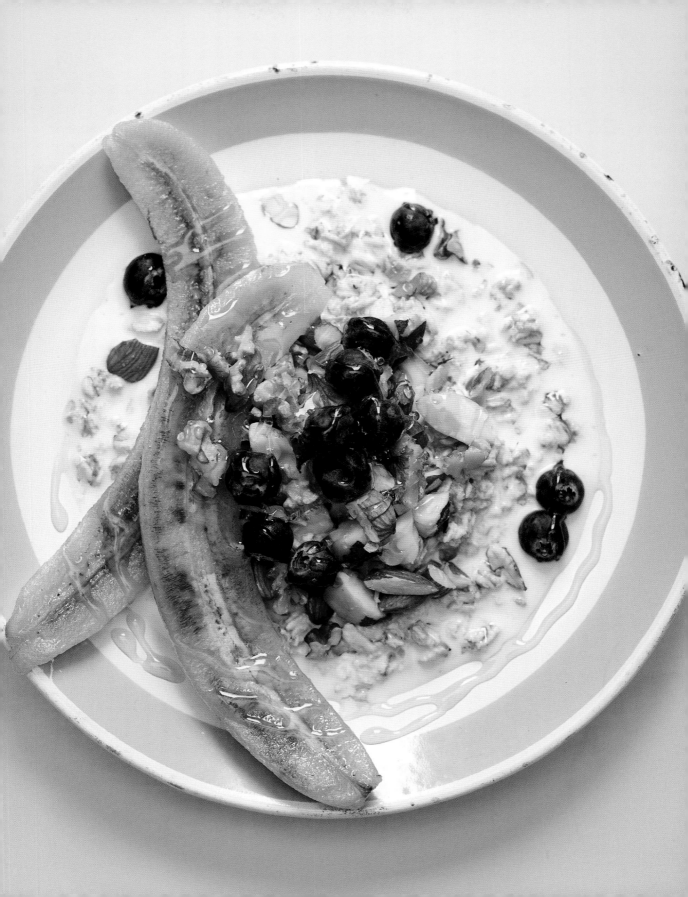

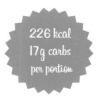

CRISPY CHICKPEA SHAKSHUKA

Instead of bread with your breakfast, why not try crispy chickpeas? They provide a delicious contrasting crunch that will take your shakshuka to the next level. Just roast them up and chuck them on top.

To make 1 portion

¼ tin of chickpeas (100g), drained

Pinch of smoked paprika for the chickpeas, plus a pinch for the shakshuka

Pinch of ground cumin for the chickpeas, plus a pinch for the shakshuka

¼ onion, sliced

¼ tin of chopped tomatoes (100g)

1 egg

Small handful of chopped coriander (optional)

Oil (any)

Salt and pepper

To cook

Preheat your oven to 180°C/gas mark 4.

Scatter the chickpeas on to a baking sheet, drizzle with oil and add a pinch each of paprika, cumin, salt and pepper. Mix well, then roast for about 25 minutes, or until nice and crispy.

Meanwhile, in a small frying pan, fry the onion in a splash of oil over a medium heat for a few minutes before adding the chopped tomatoes, along with a pinch each of paprika, cumin, salt and pepper. Simmer for about 7 minutes, then make a little well in the tomatoes and crack in the egg. Once the egg is cooked, add the crispy chickpeas, sprinkle with chopped coriander, if using, and serve.

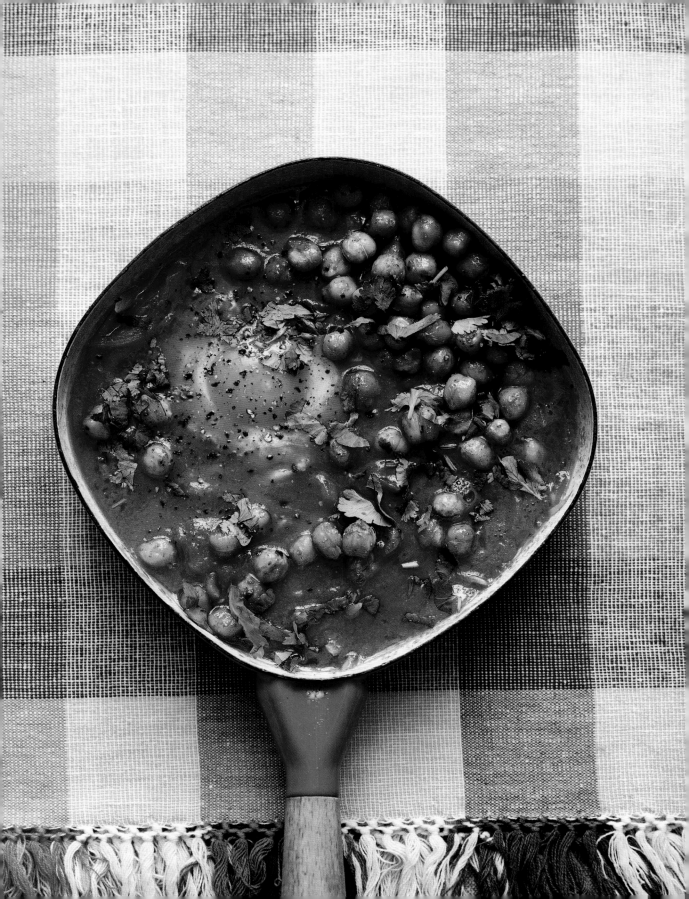

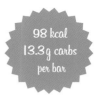

PEANUT BUTTER BREAKFAST BARS

Some so-called breakfast bars are really just desserts with a breakfast wrapping. So here, I have created a version that's packed with protein, fibre and healthy fats to keep you full up for longer – a much healthier way to start the day.

To make 8 bars

1 mug of rolled oats

Handful of raisins

2 tbsp smooth peanut butter

2 tbsp honey

1 egg

To cook

Preheat your oven to 180°C/gas mark 4 and line a small baking tin with greaseproof paper.

Mix together the oats, raisins, peanut butter, honey and egg in a bowl until well combined. Transfer the mixture to the lined tin and press down with the back of a spoon (the mixture should be about 2cm thick). Bake for about 20 minutes, then leave to cool before chopping into neat bars.

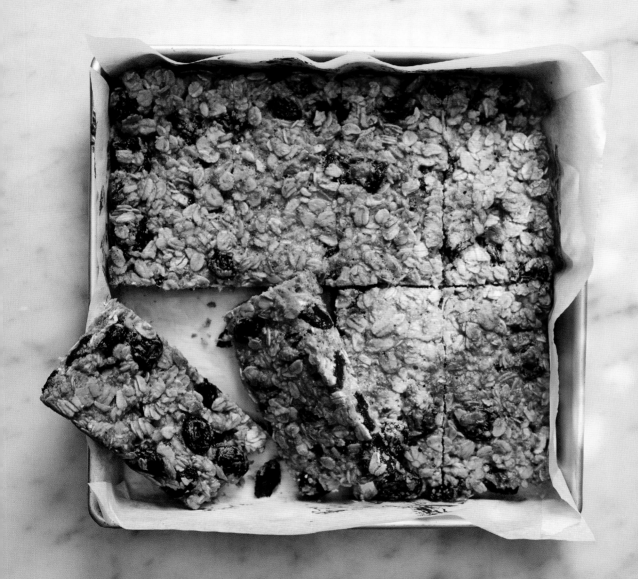

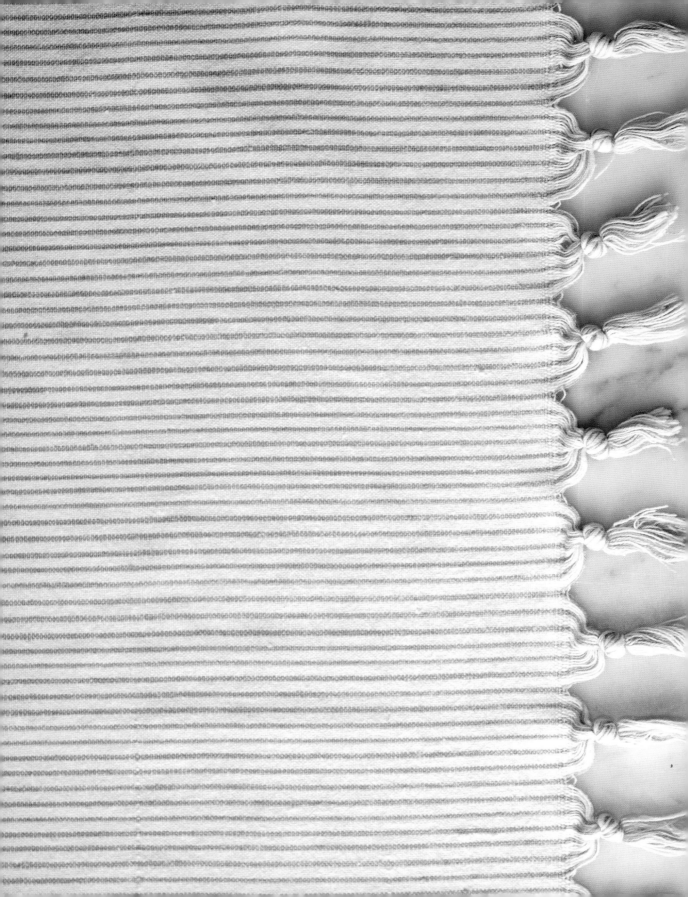

LUNCH

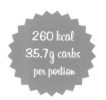

260 kcal
35.7g carbs
per portion

AUBERGINE 'BACON' BLT

Aubergine is a great lower-calorie substitute for bacon, and you can still achieve that smoky flavour with a pinch of paprika. You can cook it to your liking and get it extra crispy, just like real bacon.

To make 1 sandwich

Pinch of smoked paprika

2–3 slices of aubergine, about 5mm thick

2 slices of bread, toasted if you like

A few lettuce leaves

A few slices of tomato

1 tsp vegan mayonnaise

Splash of soy sauce

Oil (any)

Salt and pepper

To cook

Mix together the paprika, soy sauce and a splash of oil in a small bowl, then rub this marinade over the aubergine slices. Pan-fry the aubergine slices over a medium heat for about 10 minutes, turning halfway through, or for however long it takes for them to become nice and caramelised on both sides. Assemble your sandwich with bread, lettuce, tomato, the cooked aubergine slices and a squirt of mayo. Don't forget to season before serving.

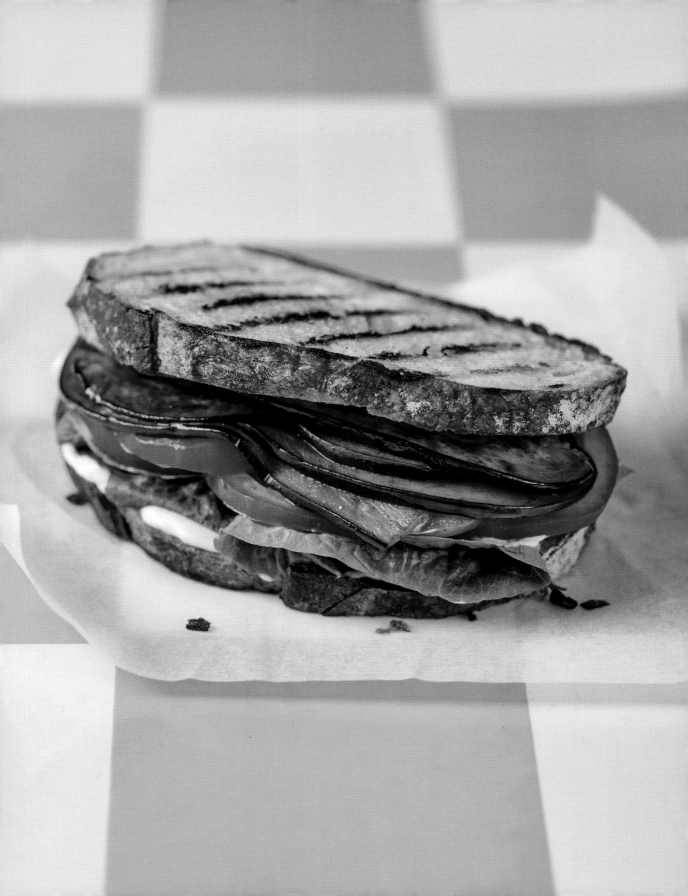

263 kcal
30.9 g carbs
per portion

POACHED EGG RAMEN

I've never understood why you can't just poach an egg in the same pan as the one you're making the soup in. It seems much more logical, but no one does it. So I thought I'd give it a go.

To make 1 portion

2 spring onions, cut into 3cm lengths

1 garlic clove, sliced

1 red chilli, seeded and sliced

A few mushrooms, sliced

½ chicken stock cube (or any stock cube)

400ml boiling water

½ pack of soft udon noodles (about 100g)

1 egg

Splash of soy sauce

Sesame oil

To cook

Pan-fry the spring onions, garlic, chilli and mushrooms in a splash of sesame oil over a medium heat for a few minutes, then crumble in the stock cube and pour in the boiling water. Add the noodles and cook for 5 minutes. Using a spoon, hold everything to one side of the pan to make a bit of room for the egg. Gently crack the egg into the space provided (if you can't crack an egg with one hand, then pre-crack it into a mug first), continuing to hold back the noodles using your spoon. After a few minutes, once the egg is cooked, serve with a splash of soy sauce.

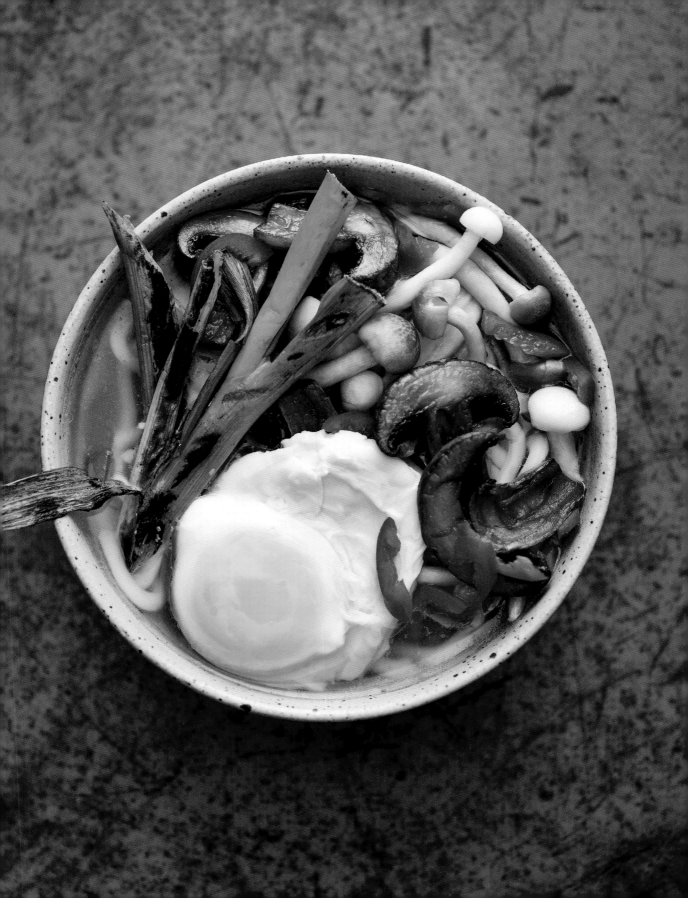

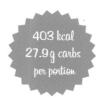

403 kcal
27.9 g carbs
per portion

AUTUMN SALAD

Often, I'm still hungry after a salad, which is annoying, so I wanted to create a more substantial option. Butternut squash is healthy and filling, plus you can also roast the seeds to add texture and nutrients to the dish. Cheese had to feature, too, so I chose a strong blue cheese because a few crumbles go a long way.

To make I portion

2–3 chunky slices of butternut squash, plus a handful of the seeds

A few lettuce leaves

Handful of walnuts, roughly chopped

Small handful of crumbled blue cheese

Drizzle of honey

Olive oil

Salt and pepper

To cook

Preheat your oven to 180°C/gas mark 4.

Place the slices of butternut squash on a baking sheet, drizzle with oil and add a pinch of salt and pepper. Roast for about 30 minutes, adding the squash seeds about halfway through.

To assemble the salad, arrange the squash slices on a bed of lettuce leaves, then add the walnuts, blue cheese and seeds. Finish with a drizzle of honey, then serve.

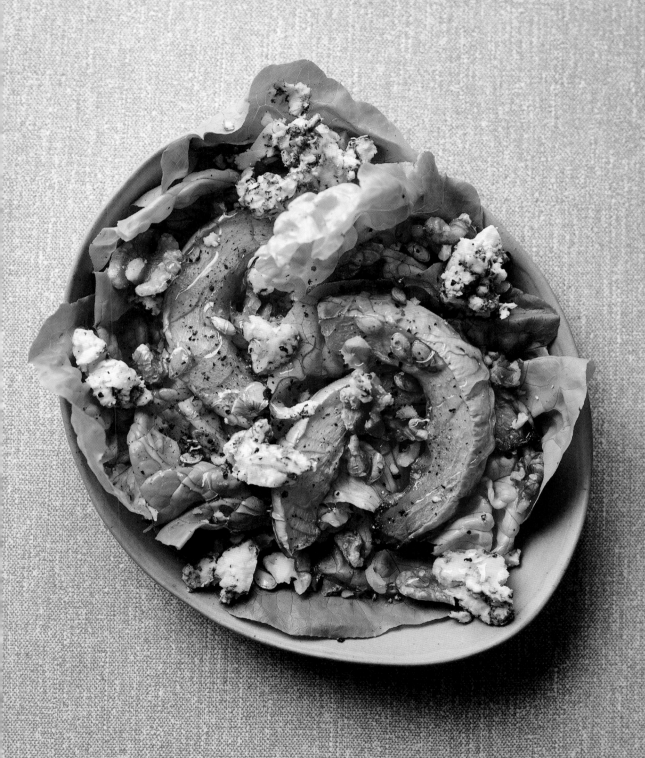

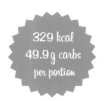

329 kcal
49.9 g carbs
per portion

HAM & MUSTARD REMOULADE TARTE

Remoulade is usually made with mayonnaise, but I've used crème fraîche for a lighter dish. Normally, I'd use buttery puff pastry, but filo has more texture (just scrunch the edges to make it lovely and crunchy) and is lower in calories.

To make 1 portion

A few sheets of filo pastry

1 slice of celeriac, cut into matchsticks

¼ apple, cut into matchsticks

1 thick slice of ham, cut into matchsticks

2 tsp crème fraîche

½ tsp wholegrain mustard (or any mustard)

Small handful of lamb's lettuce (or anything green and salady)

Oil (any)

Salt and pepper

To cook

Preheat your oven to 180°C/gas mark 4.

Slightly dampen the filo sheets with a brush of oil, then place them in an ovenproof dish and scrunch the edges. Bake in the oven for roughly 12 minutes, or until cooked and golden brown (timing will vary depending on your scrunching technique, so keep an eye out).

Meanwhile, in a bowl, mix together the celeriac, apple, ham, crème fraîche and mustard. Season to taste, then spoon into the pastry case, and top with some lamb's lettuce to serve.

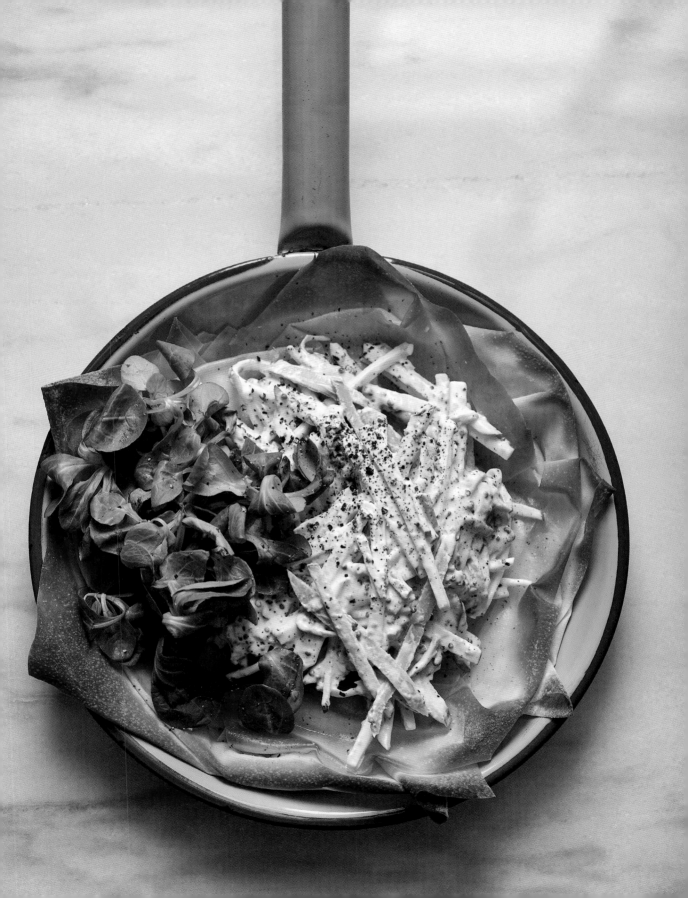

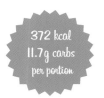

372 kcal
11.7g carbs
per portion

HALLOUMI CHOPPED SALAD

Make salads extra fun and extra tasty by using halloumi. A little goes a long way, and this chopped salad technique means it all gets mixed up nicely so you're not left with a boring last few mouthfuls. Honey and halloumi are a classic combo, so I have used a drizzle of honey in the dressing, making it taste decadent even though it's only a small amount. I have also used the juice from the tomatoes as the base for the dressing rather than oil. A great low-carb option with a summery Mediterranean vibe.

To make 1 portion

Handful of cherry tomatoes, halved

¼ block of halloumi, cut into 2.5cm cubes

A few lettuce leaves, finely chopped

½ tsp honey

½ tsp Dijon mustard

Small handful of crushed pistachios

Olive oil

Salt and pepper

To cook

Chuck the tomatoes into a bowl, then add a drizzle of olive oil, a pinch of salt and a pinch of pepper. Leave to stand for about 15 minutes while you get everything else ready.

Pan-fry the halloumi in a splash of oil over a medium–high heat for about 10 minutes until nicely coloured on all sides.

Toss together the chopped lettuce and halloumi in a bowl. Using a fork or slotted spoon, add the tomatoes, keeping their juice in the tomato bowl.

To make the dressing, mix the tomato juice with the honey and mustard, adding a little more of each if you think it needs it, then pour over the salad. Scatter over the crushed pistachios and serve.

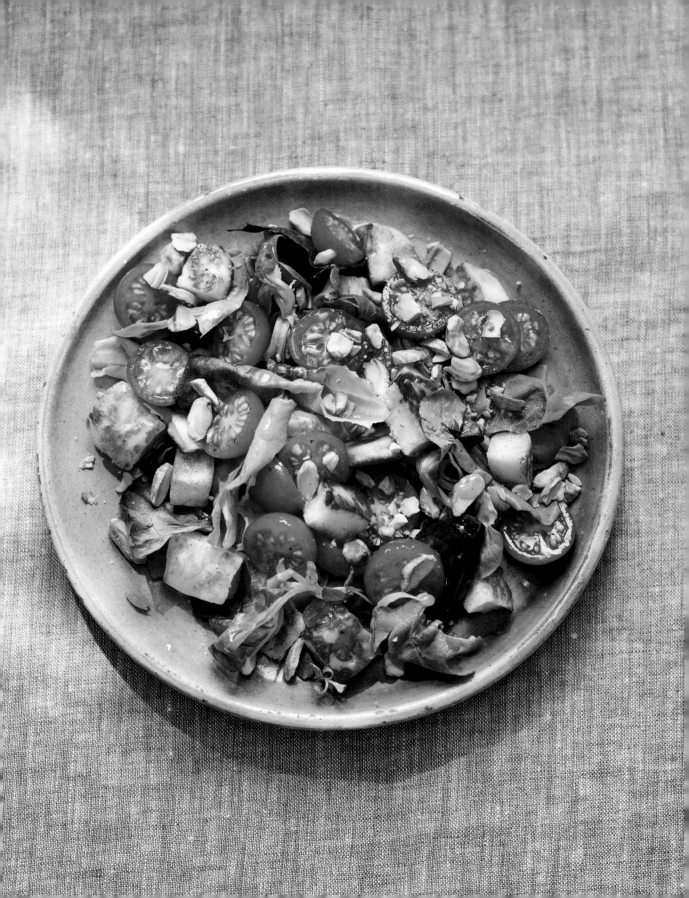

233 kcal
32.8 g carbs
per portion

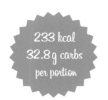

SPICED CARROT & LENTIL SOUP

I like to make soup more filling by adding lentils. This is a substantial main meal that keeps me full – no bread roll required.

To make 1 portion

½ onion, diced

1 tsp cumin seeds

½ tsp curry powder

Pinch of dried chilli flakes

1 large carrot, diced

Small handful of dried red split lentils

½ vegetable stock cube

400ml water

Dollop of crème fraîche (optional)

Oil (any)

Salt and pepper

To cook

Pan-fry the onion in a splash of oil over a medium heat for about 5 minutes until softened. Add the cumin seeds, curry powder, chilli flakes and a pinch of salt and pepper and continue to fry for a few more minutes. Remove a teaspoon of the mixture and set to one side to be used as a garnish later, then add the diced carrot and lentils. Crumble in the stock cube and pour in the water. Simmer for 20 minutes, adding more water if required, then blend with a hand-held stick blender until smooth.

Serve topped with a dollop of crème fraîche, if using, and the reserved onion and cumin seed mixture sprinkled over.

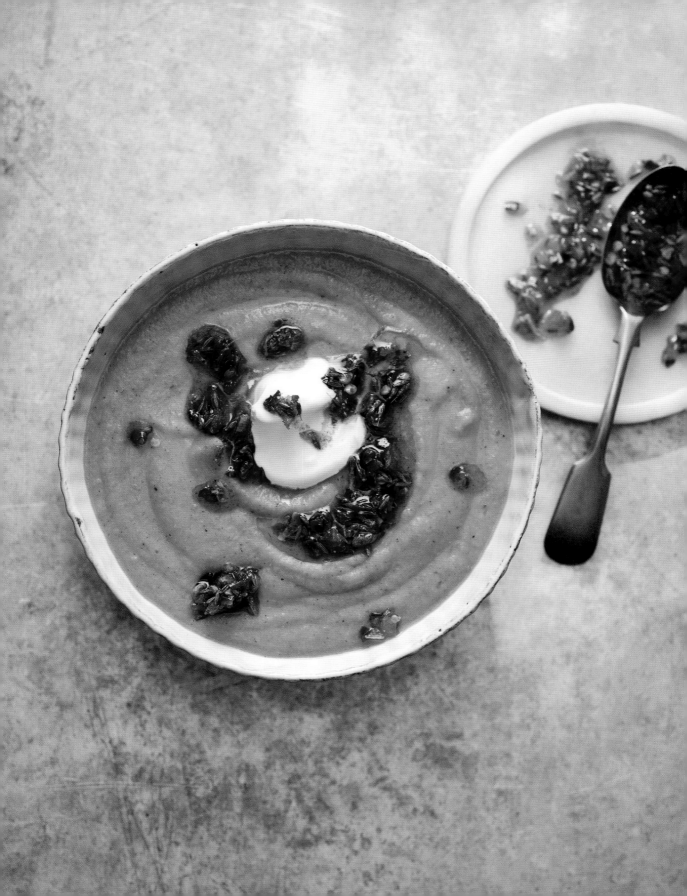

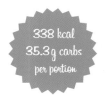

338 kcal
35.3g carbs
per portion

CHORIZO-STUFFED RED PEPPERS

Chorizo has such a powerful flavour that you only need a small amount for the dish to taste amazing. I like to use this to my advantage – it is one of the cornerstones of One Pound Meals, as well as a great philosophy for healthy eating on the cheap.

To make 1 stuffed pepper

Small handful of cubed chorizo

1 spring onion, sliced

½ tsp tomato purée

Handful of leftover cooked rice

1 red pepper

Small handful of chopped parsley (optional)

Oil (any)

Salt and pepper

To cook

Preheat your oven to 180°C/gas mark 4.

Pan-fry the chorizo and spring onion in a dry frying pan over a medium heat for a few minutes. Add the tomato purée and continue cooking for another minute, then add the cooked rice and seasoning, and mix everything together.

Cut the top off the pepper, scrape out the seeds, then fill it with the rice mixture, put the top back on and bake for about 20 minutes on a baking tray. Once cooked, garnish with chopped parsley, if using, and serve.

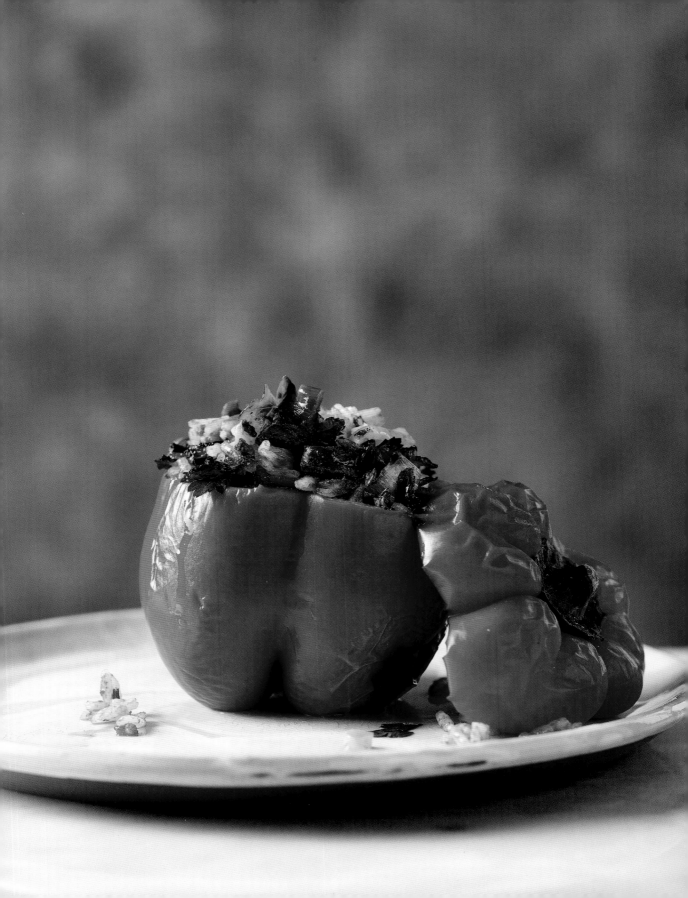

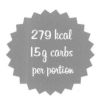

279 kcal
15g carbs
per portion

BEETROOT SALAD

When you use beetroot as the main ingredient for a salad, you don't really need a dressing because it's so flavoursome. This is great news, because it means the dish is much lower in calories – so, give this a try and see what you think.

To make 1 portion

2 pre-cooked beetroots, thinly sliced

Handful of rocket

Handful of crumbled feta

Handful of walnuts, roughly chopped

Salt and pepper

To prepare

Arrange the beetroot slices on a plate. Top with the rocket, feta and walnuts. Season lightly, then serve.

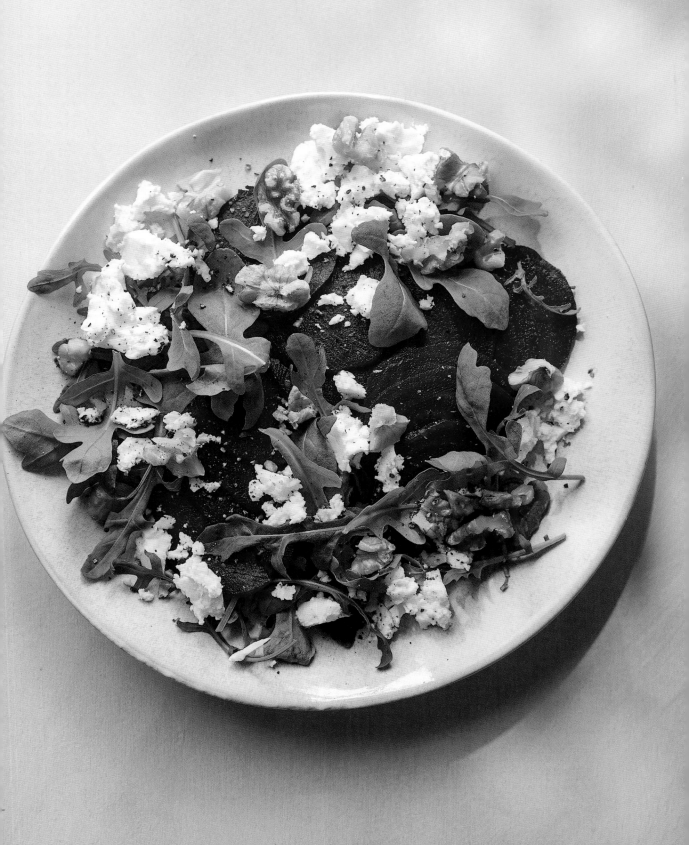

OVEN BHAJIS

Instead of deep-frying these bhajis in lots of oil, I've created a healthier oven-baked alternative for you to try. Serve with your favourite dip.

To make 1 portion (3 bhajis)

1 onion, sliced

Small handful of chopped coriander

½ carrot, cut into matchsticks

2 tbsp gram flour (chickpea flour)

Pinch of curry powder

Salt and pepper

To cook

Preheat your oven to 180°C/gas mark 4 and line a baking sheet with greaseproof paper.

Mix together the onion, coriander, carrot, gram flour and curry powder in a bowl. Season with salt and pepper, then add a little water splash by splash, while mixing, until it all sticks together.

Divide into 3 portions on the lined baking tray and shape into bhajis. Bake for about 15–20 minutes until cooked through and nicely coloured.

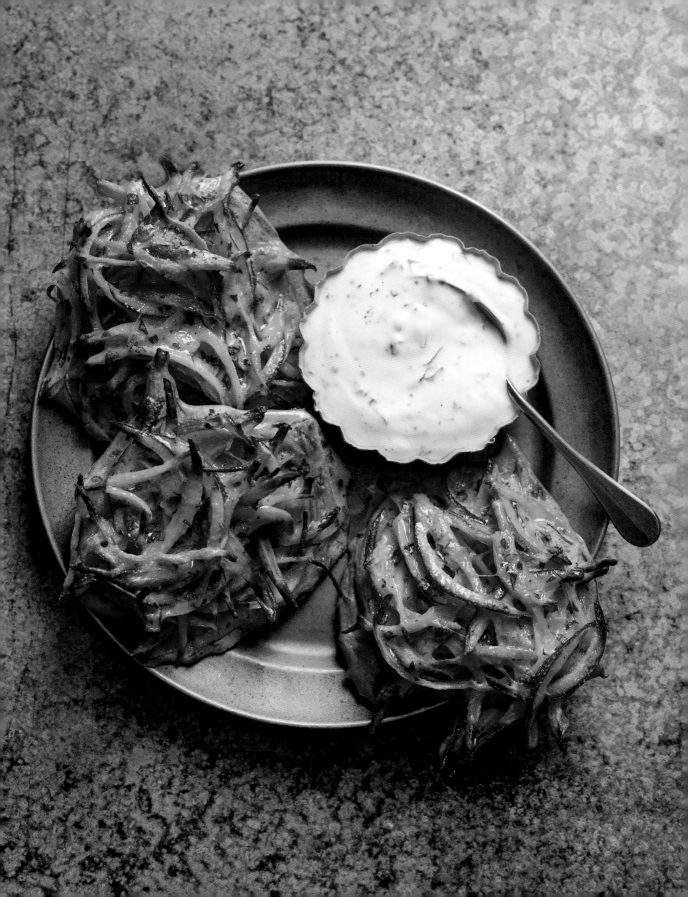

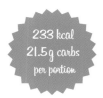

233 kcal
21.5g carbs
per portion

GREEK POTATO SALAD

Usually, potato salad contains a lot of mayo, so I thought it would be a nice idea to try feta to bring it together instead. It's even more delicious – plus it's a well-balanced and super-healthy meal.

To make 1 portion

Handful of baby potatoes, halved

A few slices of red onion

Handful of feta cubes

Handful of pitted black olives

Handful of chopped parsley

Squeeze of lemon juice

Olive oil

Salt and pepper

To cook

Start by boiling the potatoes for about 15 minutes, or until cooked through. Drain and leave to cool slightly.

Tip the still-warm potatoes into a bowl, then add the red onion, feta, black olives and chopped parsley. Season to taste and finish with a drizzle of olive oil and a squeeze of lemon.

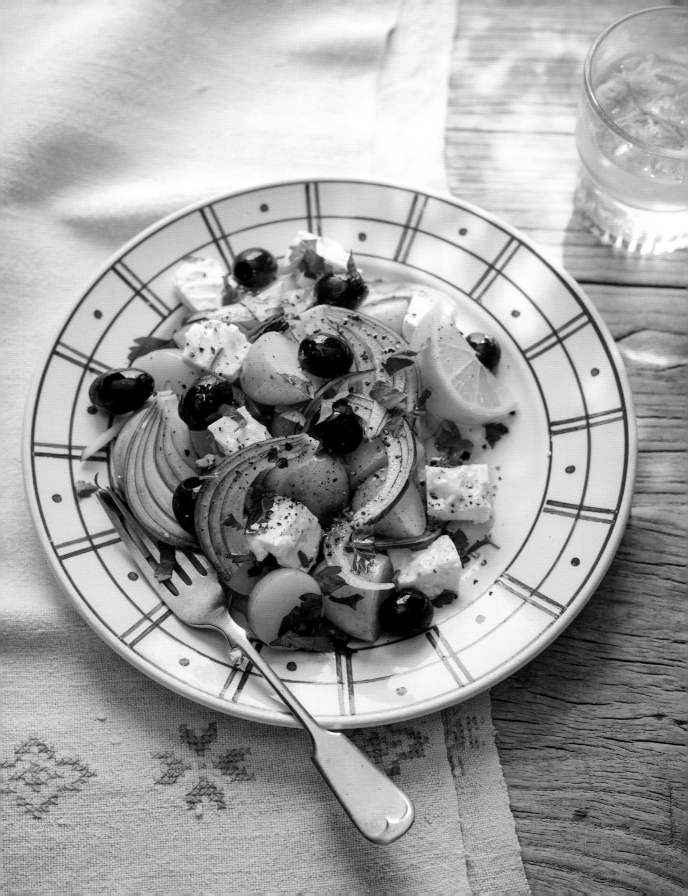

258 kcal
3.3g carbs
per portion

SAVOY CABBAGE EGG

This is a bit like a cross between a spring roll and an omelette. Don't be scared to get a bit of caramelisation on the cabbage, because it will add to the flavour.

To make 1 portion

Handful of shredded savoy cabbage

1 garlic clove, sliced

3 eggs, beaten

Splash of soy sauce

Sesame oil

Salt and pepper

To cook

Season the cabbage and pan-fry in a splash of sesame oil over a high heat for a couple of minutes before adding the garlic and cooking for a further couple of minutes. Remove from the pan and set aside. Reduce the heat to medium and add the beaten eggs, tilting the pan so they spread out evenly. Leave to cook for 30 seconds, or until they're about 25% done, then pile the cabbage on top and add a splash of soy sauce. Carry on cooking for another minute or so until the eggs are cooked through, then serve.

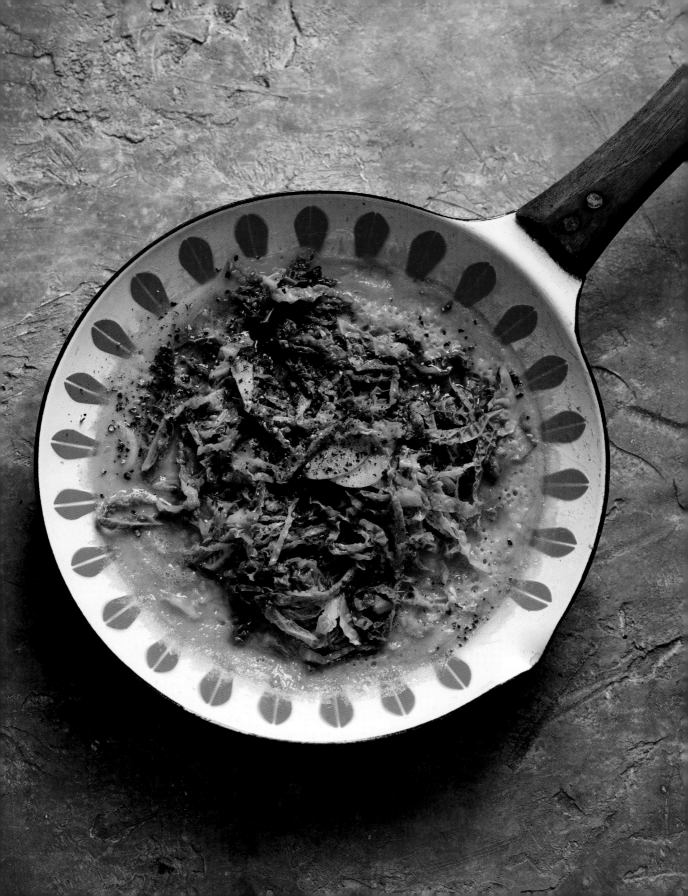

132 kcal
12.7 g carbs
per portion

BAKED CORN RIBS

Corn ribs have become hugely popular in restaurants over the past few years, but they are almost always deep-fried. Fortunately, you can also bake them for a healthier version – the tastiest baked veg you'll ever eat. So, if you're unfamiliar with this new trend, give these a try – they are well worth it.

To make 1 portion

1 sweetcorn cob

½ tsp paprika, plus a pinch to garnish

Pinch of chopped parsley

Pinch of dried chilli flakes

Lime wedge

Oil (any)

Salt and pepper

To cook

Preheat your oven to its highest temperature and line a baking tray with baking parchment.

Very carefully chop your corn in half lengthways and then chop each half lengthways again, and repeat once more. Please be careful; this is without doubt THE MOST DANGEROUS thing I've ever done in the kitchen. If in doubt, give it a google and see the technique. Some people bash the knife with a rolling pin, some lean on it – just do whatever you feel is safest.

Once cut, drizzle with oil, add paprika, salt and pepper, then mix together to coat evenly. Arrange on the prepared tray, then roast in the oven for about 30 minutes until cooked and slightly charred. Finish with a sprinkling of chopped parsley, a pinch of chilli flakes, a pinch of paprika and a squeeze of lime.

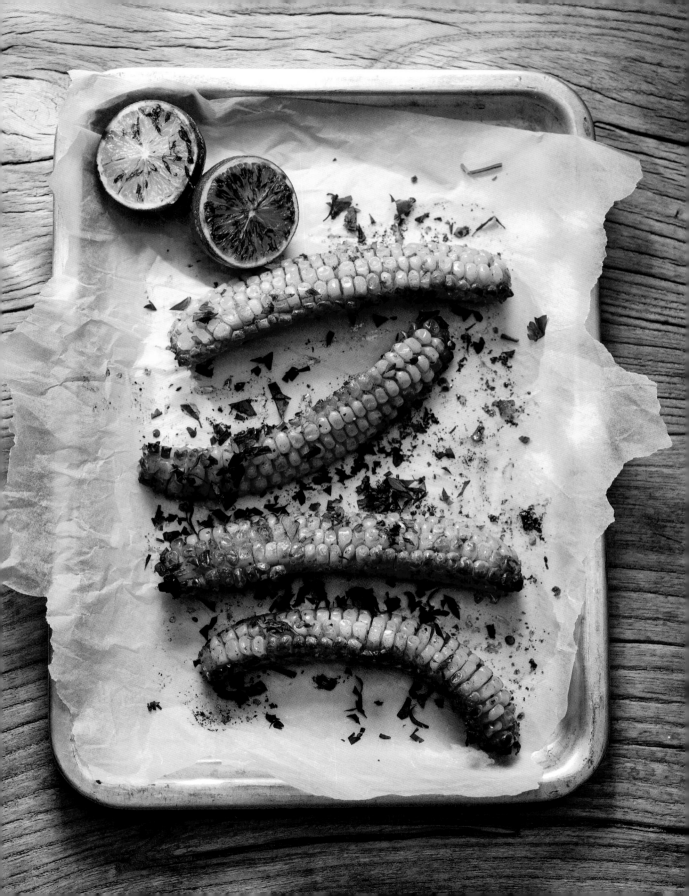

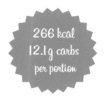

266 kcal
12.1 g carbs
per portion

TOFU ALMONDINE

Inspiration can come from anywhere. I once read an interview with Jeremy Strong where he was eating trout almondine in a restaurant in Williamsburg. For weeks I kept thinking about it, and eventually I came up with my own budget version using tofu. Turns out this is actually a clever little low-carb recipe.

To make 1 portion

Small handful of flaked almonds

1 tbsp plain flour

1 slice of tofu, about 2.5cm thick

Handful of green beans

Squeeze of lemon juice

¼ tsp Dijon mustard

Small handful of chopped parsley

Oil (any)

Salt and pepper

To cook

Toast the almonds in a dry pan over a medium–high heat for a few minutes until lightly coloured, then remove from the pan and set aside. Season the flour and use it to coat the tofu. Add some oil to the pan and cook the tofu and green beans for about 5 minutes on each side, or until the beans are cooked and the tofu is nicely coloured.

In a bowl, combine the almonds with a squeeze of lemon juice, the Dijon mustard, the chopped parsley and a splash of water. Spoon over the tofu and beans and serve.

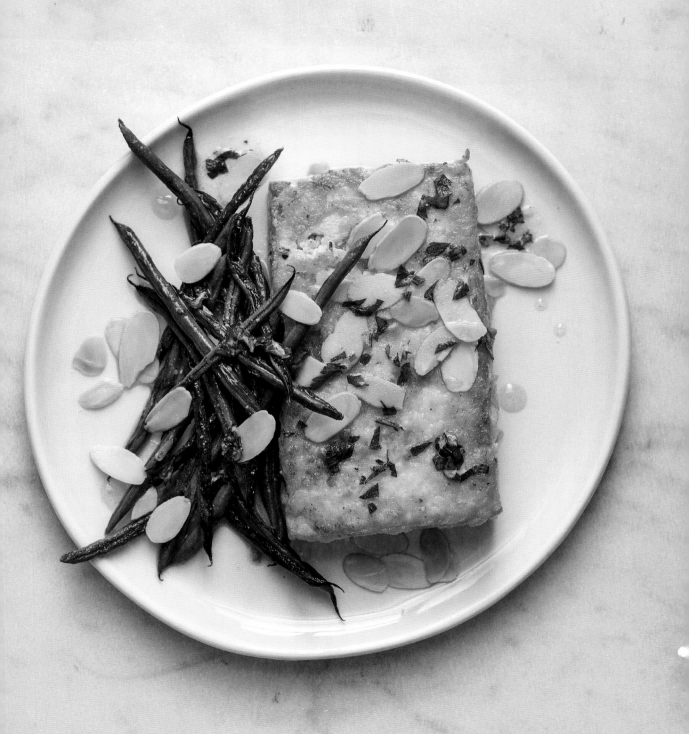

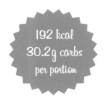
192 kcal
30.2g carbs
per portion

CREAMY PUMPKIN SOUP WITH SAGE CROUTONS

You can totally substitute pumpkin with butternut squash here if you like. Both pumpkin and butternut squash have a lovely velvety texture, so this soup feels luxurious even without the addition of cream.

To make 1 portion

Big handful of cubed pumpkin (or butternut squash)

½ onion

1 garlic clove, peeled but left whole

A few chunks of stale bread

A few sage leaves, roughly chopped

½ vegetable stock cube

Boiling water

Olive Oil

Salt and pepper

To cook

Preheat your oven to 180°C/gas mark 4.

Place the cubed pumpkin, onion and garlic on a baking sheet. Drizzle with olive oil and season. Roast for about 20 minutes until everything is soft and cooked. This will depend on their relative sizes, so you might have to remove some things earlier.

Meanwhile, scatter the chunks of bread on to a separate baking sheet, then drizzle with oil and sprinkle with salt, pepper and the chopped sage. When the pumpkin has been in the oven for 10 minutes, add the croutons and cook for 10 minutes until nicely toasted.

Throw the roasted pumpkin, onion and garlic into a blender, then crumble in the stock cube and pour in a splash of boiling water from the kettle. Blend and keep adding water until you get your desired consistency.

Serve the soup with the croutons on top.

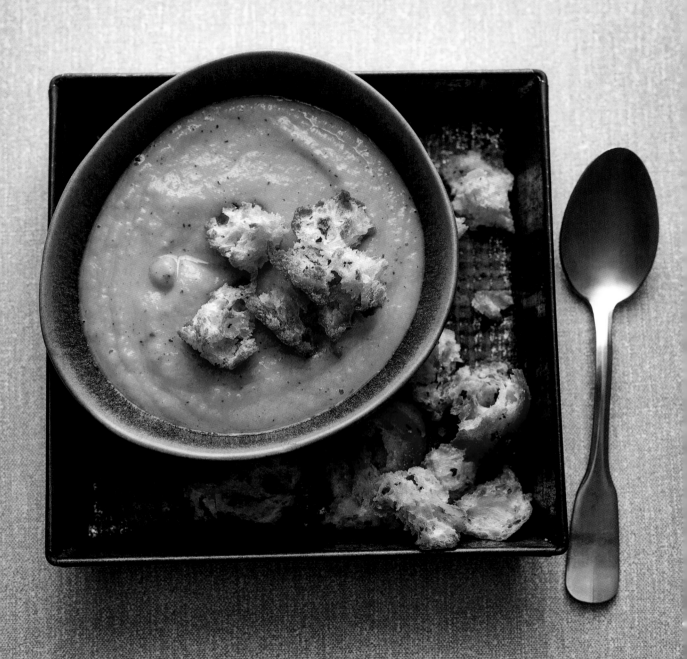

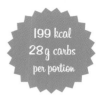

CRISPY MUSHROOM PANCAKES

Here, mushrooms are a delicious alternative to duck. Not only are they cheaper, they're also much lower in calories – but they're still really satisfying. If you want that meaty crispiness, then I'd go for a king oyster mushroom but feel free to use whatever you've got. To make it even cheaper, you could even make your own wraps by mixing 40g of plain flour with 25g of water, kneading, dividing into 3, rolling out with a rolling pin and cooking in a dry pan for about 30 seconds on each side.

To make 1 portion

½ tsp Chinese 5-spice

2 king oyster mushrooms, shredded with a fork

2 Chinese pancakes

2 tsp hoisin sauce

1 spring onion, sliced into matchsticks

2.5cm piece cucumber, sliced into matchsticks

Oil (any)

Salt and pepper

To cook

In a bowl, mix a splash of oil with the Chinese 5-spice and a pinch of salt and pepper. Add the shredded mushrooms and mix well.

Pan-fry over a medium heat for about 10–15 minutes until dark in colour and crispy.

Meanwhile, warm the pancakes in a microwave or oven as per the instructions on the packet.

To serve, place a dollop of hoisin sauce on to each pancake, then top with the crispy mushrooms, sliced spring onions and cucumber.

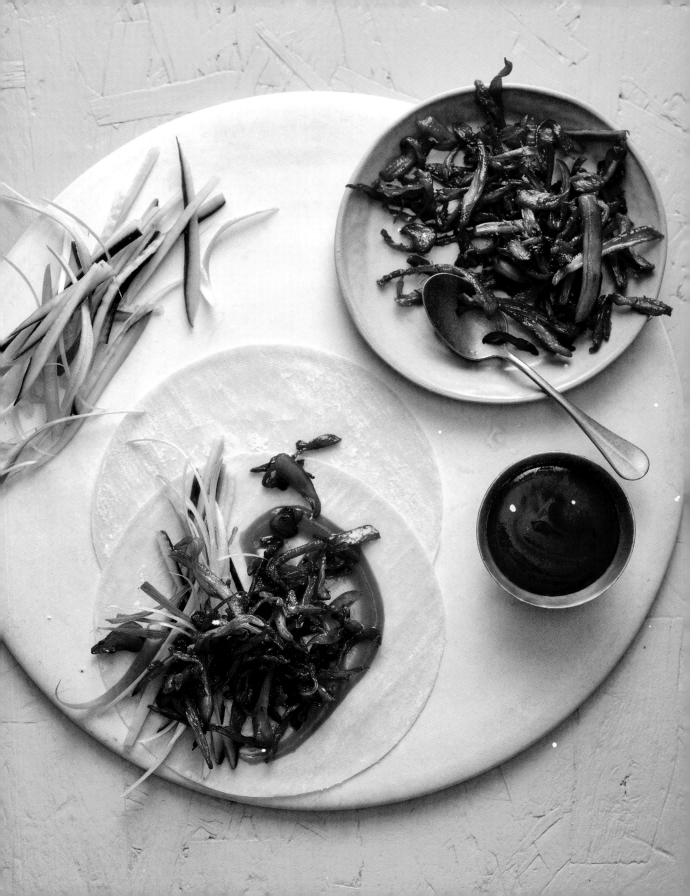

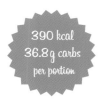

390 kcal
36.8g carbs
per portion

THE RACHEL SALAD

This salad went viral when it was alleged that Jennifer Aniston ate it every day on the set of *Friends*. She recently clarified that this wasn't actually true, but I had already fallen in love with it, so it'll always be The Rachel Salad to me.

I did make one major adjustment, though: I took out the chickpeas, because I'm just not a fan of chickpeas straight out of the tin in a salad; I feel they need a bit more care and attention. This is a fresh, nutritious and well-balanced meal – and, most importantly, it's delicious enough to eat every day on the set of a hit sitcom.

To make 1 portion

Handful of bulgur wheat

Small handful of diced cucumber

Small handful of diced red onion

Small handful of crumbled feta cheese

Small handful of pistachios

Small handful of chopped parsley

Small handful of chopped mint

Squeeze of lemon juice

Olive oil

Salt and pepper

To cook

Cook the bulgur wheat in plenty of salted boiling water for 15 minutes, then drain and allow to cool. Tip the cooked bulgur wheat into a bowl, and add the cucumber, red onion, feta, pistachios, parsley and mint. Add a generous glug of olive oil and a squeeze of lemon juice, then season to taste before serving.

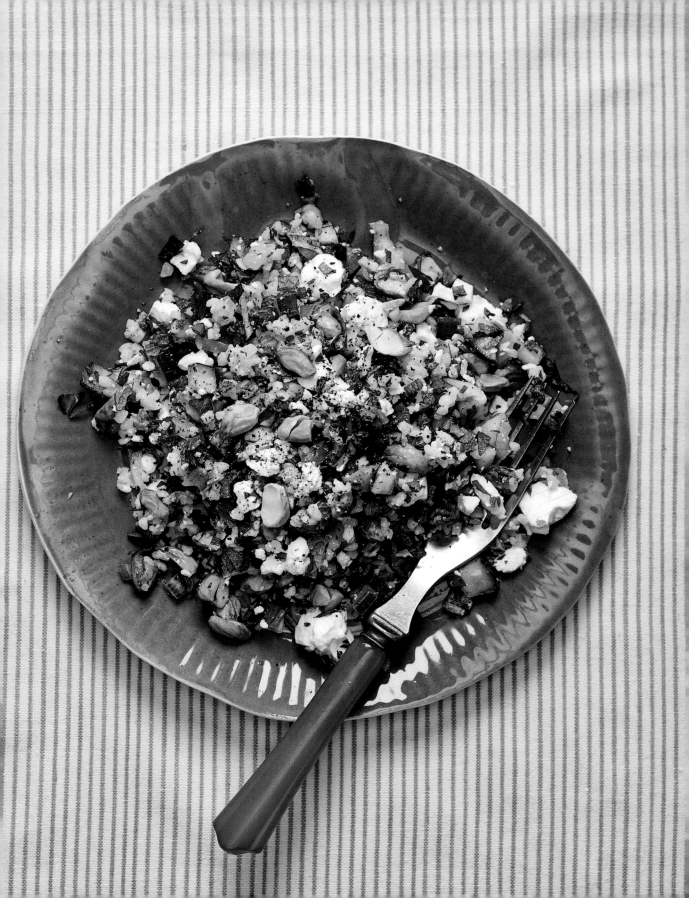

112 kcal
5.3g carbs
per portion

AUBERGINE PIZZETTE

Do you have half an aubergine left over from the Oven Aubergine Schnitzel recipe on page 188? Well, try this! It's a variation on a pizza, but without the carb-heavy base. Aubergines are so versatile and so tasty that you should definitely add them to your shopping list.

To make 1 pizzette

½ aubergine, cut into 3 slices

Pinch of dried oregano for the base, plus a pinch for the topping

¼ tin of chopped tomatoes (100g)

¼ mozzarella ball

A few basil leaves (optional)

Salt and pepper

To cook

Preheat your oven to 180°C/gas mark 4.

Place the aubergine on a baking sheet, skin-side down. Sprinkle with a pinch each of salt, pepper and oregano, then bake for about 15 minutes. Top with the tomato and mozzarella, then sprinkle over a little more salt and pepper, and another pinch of oregano. Bake for about 20 minutes until the cheese is bubbling, then garnish with basil, if using, and serve.

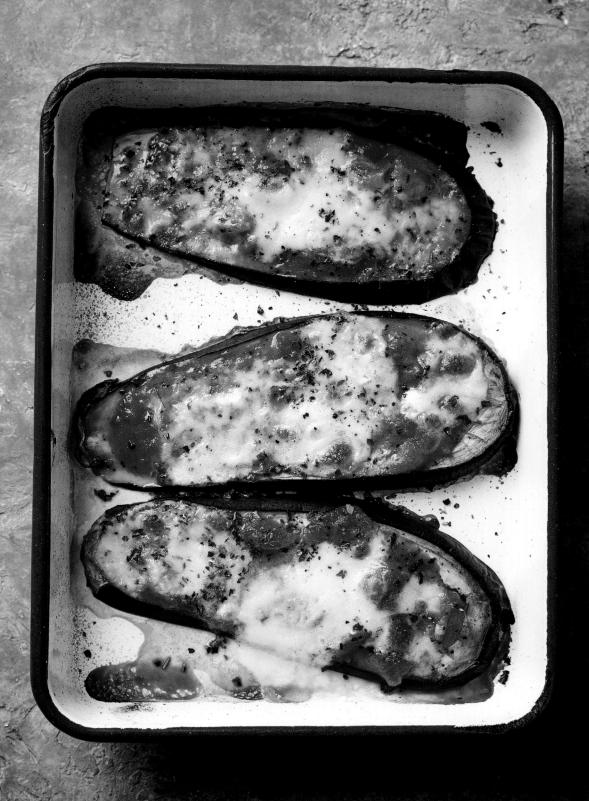

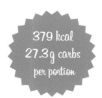
379 kcal
27.3g carbs
per portion

BAKED ZUCCHINI BALLS

I've called these 'zucchini balls' because it sounds more like something they'd eat in *The Sopranos* than 'courgette balls', and that was the vibe I was aiming for. They are like a lower-calorie meatball, but equally delicious.

To make 1 portion

1 courgette

1 tbsp plain flour

1 egg

Small handful of grated Parmesan, plus extra to garnish

Small handful of breadcrumbs

Pinch of dried oregano for the balls, plus a pinch for the sauce

1 garlic clove, sliced

½ tin of chopped tomatoes (200g)

Oil (any)

Salt and pepper

To cook

Preheat your oven to 180°C/gas mark 4 and line a baking tray with baking parchment.

Grate the courgette into a colander, then add a pinch of salt and allow to sit for 20 minutes to draw out the water. Push down on the courgette with the back of a spoon to squeeze out as much water as possible, then transfer to a bowl along with the flour, egg, Parmesan and breadcrumbs. Season with salt, pepper and a pinch of oregano and mix well. Roll the mixture into roughly 8 balls. Place on the prepared baking tray, then brush with oil and bake for about 20 minutes until lightly coloured.

Meanwhile, pan-fry the garlic in a splash of oil over a medium heat for a few minutes, just until it starts to colour, then add the chopped tomatoes and simmer for about 12 minutes. Season to taste and add a splash of water if it becomes too thick.

Add the cooked courgette balls to the sauce and serve with an extra sprinkle of Parmesan and some black pepper.

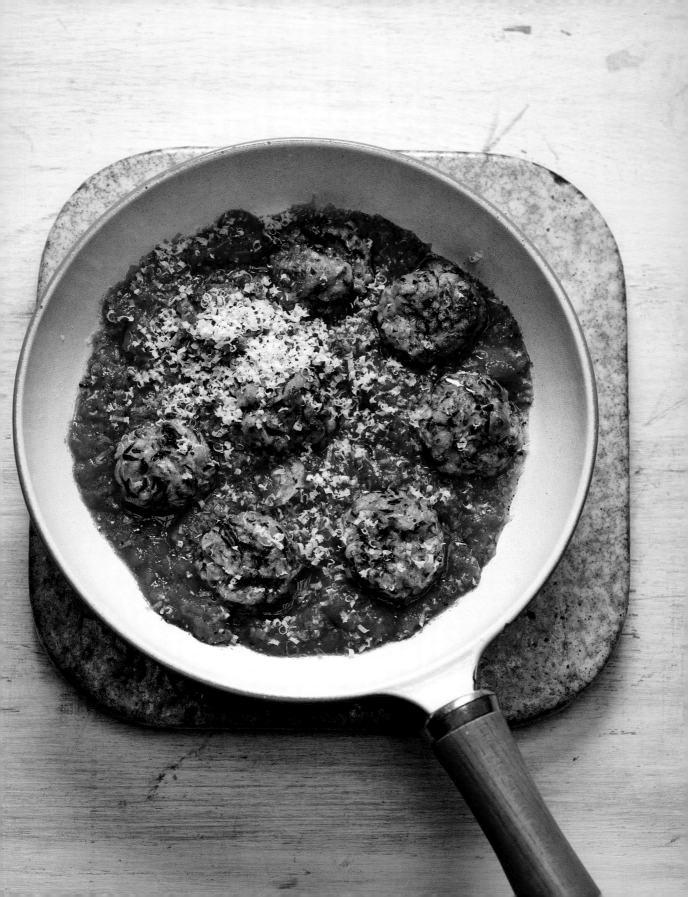

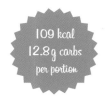

OVEN-ROASTED TOMATO SOUP

If you want to boost the flavour of tomatoes, then simply roast them with salt, pepper and oregano. Something magical happens. So, I thought, why not make them into the best tomato soup ever?

To make 1 portion

½ onion, sliced

2 garlic cloves, halved lengthways

Big handful of cherry tomatoes, halved

½ tsp dried oregano

Boiling water

Oil (any)

Salt and pepper

To cook

Preheat your oven to 180°C/gas mark 4.

Lay the sliced onions and garlic on a baking sheet, then arrange the tomatoes on top. Drizzle with oil and season with salt, pepper and oregano. Roast for about 25 minutes, or until you start to see some caramelisation (timings will vary, so keep an eye on it).

Chuck it all into a blender and blend, then pour in some boiling water from the kettle, adding it bit by bit until you get the desired consistency. Season to taste and serve.

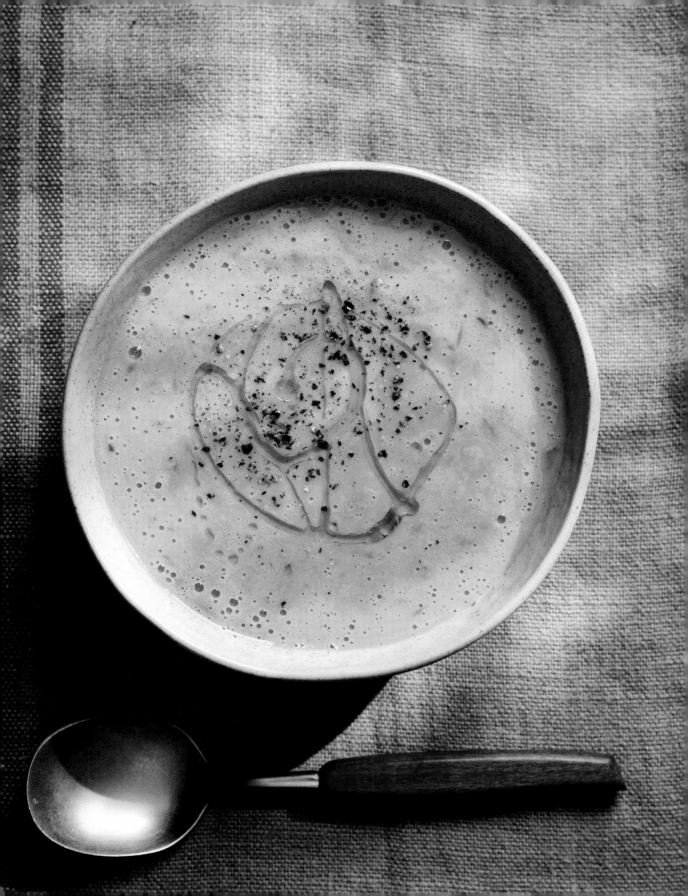

333 kcal
42.2 g carbs
per portion

TEXAN SALSA SALAD

This salsa is a substantial affair, chock-full of veg. The measurements are not important here; just chuck everything in by the handful. If you want to use a single type of bean instead of mixed beans, then kidney beans and haricot beans both work great. The addition of beans makes this salad especially high in fibre, plus you can leave out the tortilla chips for a lower-calorie option.

To make 1 portion

Small handful of tinned sweetcorn, drained

Small handful of diced green peppers

Small handful of tinned mixed beans, drained

Small handful of diced tomato

Small handful of diced red onion

Small handful of chopped coriander (optional)

2 tbsp red wine vinegar

Squeeze of lime juice

Handful of tortilla chips

Olive oil

Salt and pepper

To prepare

Put the sweetcorn, green peppers, beans, tomato, red onion and coriander, if using, into a bowl. Next add a generous glug of olive oil, the red wine vinegar and a squeeze of lime juice. Mix everything together, season to taste and serve with tortilla chips.

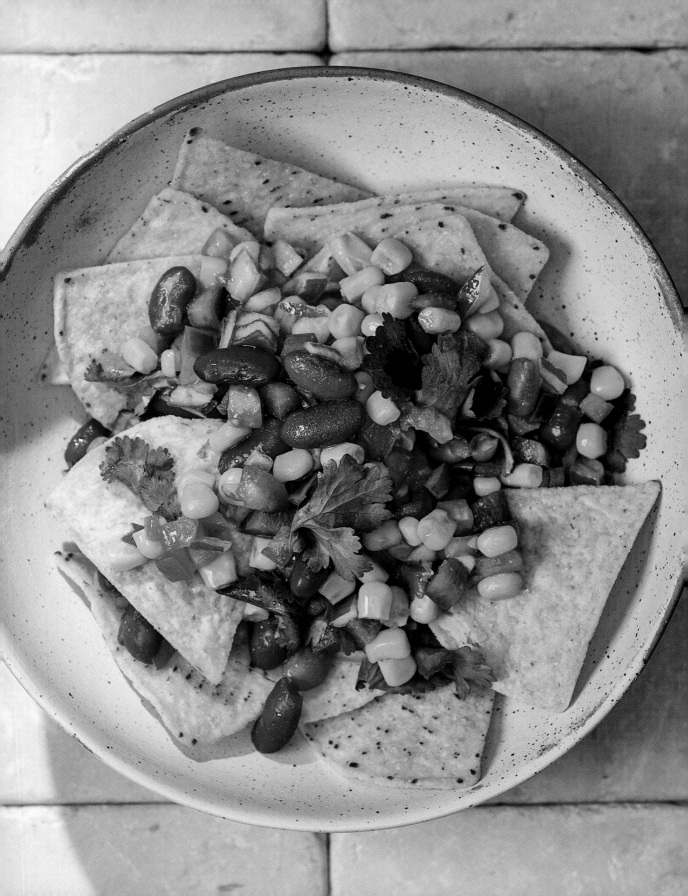

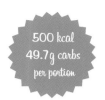

FILO PASTRY BROCCOLI TART

Filo pastry is a lower-calorie alternative to puff pastry. It may be less buttery, but it has a wonderful texture and an audible crunch when you bite into it. The key to this dish is to cut the Tenderstem broccoli lengthways so the stalks are thin enough and cook quickly.

To make 2 portions

2 sheets of filo pastry

2 tbsp vegetarian pesto

A few spears of Tenderstem broccoli, sliced lengthways

Small handful of crumbled feta

Oil (any)

Salt and pepper

To cook

Preheat your oven to 180°C/gas mark 4.

Lay your sheets of pastry one on top of the other in a rectangular dish, then scrunch up the edges. Lightly brush the edges with oil and spread the pesto over the base using the back of a spoon. Arrange the broccoli pieces over the pesto and brush with oil. Season, then bake in the oven for about 10–15 minutes, or until the edges of the tart are golden brown and the broccoli is cooked. Finish with a sprinkle of crumbled feta, some more black pepper, and serve.

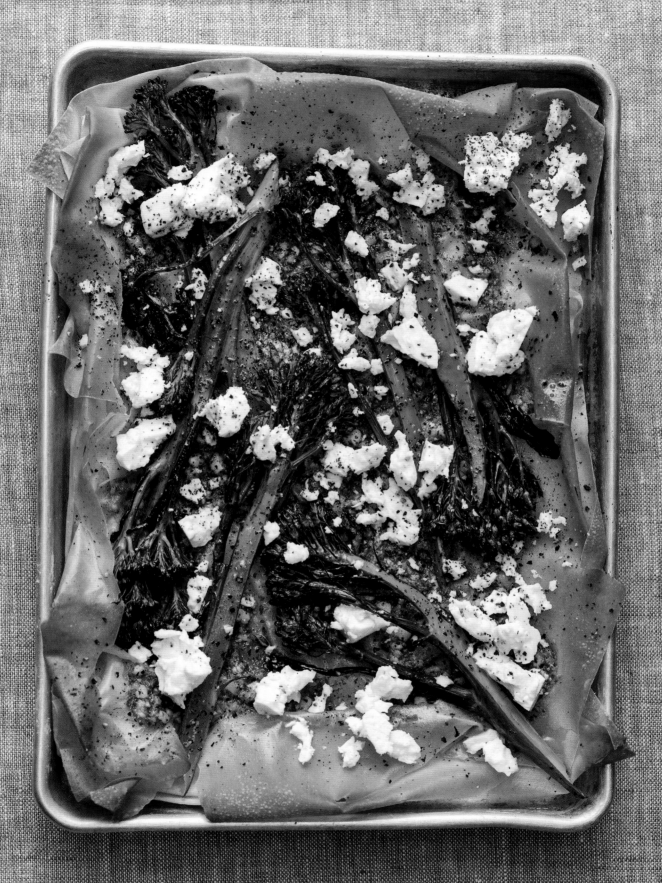

359 kcal
51.9 g carbs
per portion

POACHED CHICKEN NOODLE SOUP

Adding noodles to an already-substantial chicken soup makes a hearty lunch that will keep you going all day. Don't be scared that you won't be full up; this isn't a light soup! All cooked in one pan, it doesn't get much easier than this.

To make 1 portion

500ml water

1 chicken stock cube

2 chicken breast mini fillets

1 carrot, roughly chopped

Small handful of frozen peas

Sheet of dried rice noodles (about 50g)

1 tsp Dijon mustard

Salt and pepper

To cook

Bring the water to the boil in a saucepan, then crumble in the stock cube. Add the chicken and carrot. Simmer for about 15 minutes until the chicken is cooked through, adding the peas and noodles for the last few minutes. Remove the chicken and shred it using two forks, then return it to the soup. Season to taste and serve with a dollop of mustard to spice it up a bit.

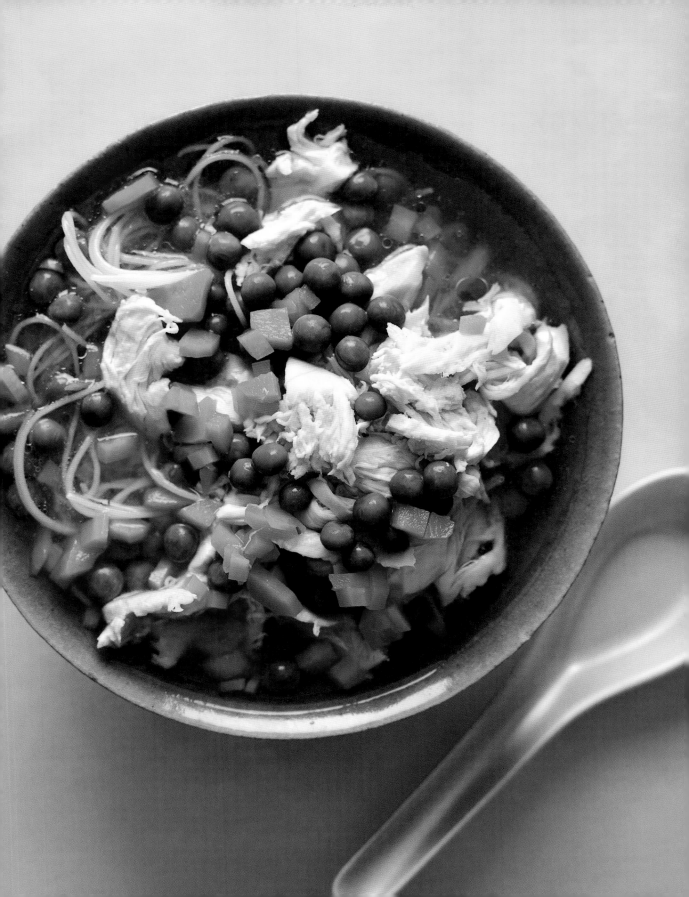

LEMON BROCCOLI COUSCOUS BOWL

422 kcal
34.1 g carbs
per portion

All my favourite flavours cooked in one pan. This is great for leftovers – a tasty, healthy and filling option for your packed lunch.

To make 1 portion

A few pieces of Tenderstem broccoli, halved lengthways

Pinch of dried chilli flakes

Small handful of pine nuts

¼ mug of couscous

¼ mug of boiling water

Squeeze of lemon, plus some grated zest

Small handful of crumbled feta cheese

Oil (any)

Salt and pepper

To cook

Pan-fry the broccoli in a splash of oil over a high heat, along with the chilli flakes, pine nuts and some salt and pepper. After about 8 minutes, once the broccoli is charred and cooked through (but still has some bite to it), remove it from the pan and set aside. With the pan off the heat, add the couscous and water, along with a squeeze of lemon. Mix together so the couscous mops up all the flavours and seasoning left in the pan, and leave for a few minutes to plump up. Fluff the couscous with a fork and spoon it on to a plate. Top with the broccoli, grate over some lemon zest and finish with some crumbled feta.

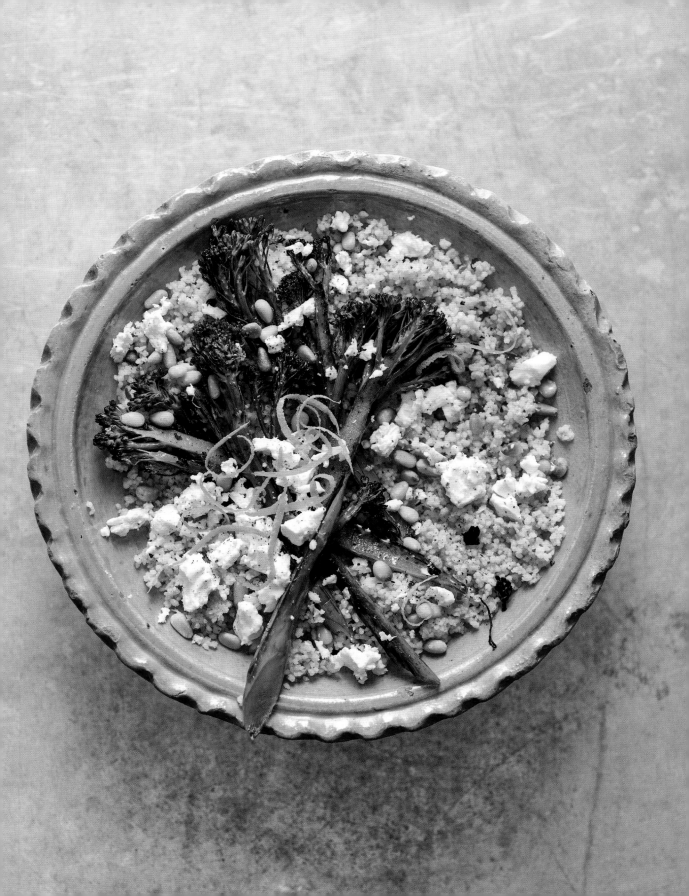

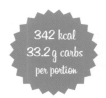

YOGHURT CAESAR SALAD

It's always a good idea to have a go-to healthy version of a Caesar dressing. You can use this on anything, not just chicken salads; you could even dip chips into it instead of mayonnaise or aioli.

To make 1 portion

½ take-and-bake ciabatta, cut into chunks

Pinch of dried oregano for the croutons, plus a pinch for the dressing

2 tbsp Greek-style yoghurt

Lemon wedge

½ garlic clove, grated

½ tsp Dijon mustard

1 tsp grated Parmesan, plus extra for garnish

A few romaine lettuce leaves, chopped

Olive oil

Salt and pepper

To cook

Preheat your oven to 180°C/gas mark 4.

Scatter the ciabatta on to a baking sheet, then drizzle with olive oil and season with salt, pepper and oregano. Bake for about 10–15 minutes until golden brown.

Meanwhile, make the dressing by mixing together the yoghurt, a squeeze of lemon juice, the garlic, the mustard, the Parmesan and a splash of water in a bowl. Season to taste with salt, pepper and oregano. If the dressing is a bit thick, loosen it with another splash of water.

Put the lettuce into a bowl, then spoon over the dressing and mix well. Sprinkle the croutons on top and finish with a little more grated Parmesan and cracked black pepper.

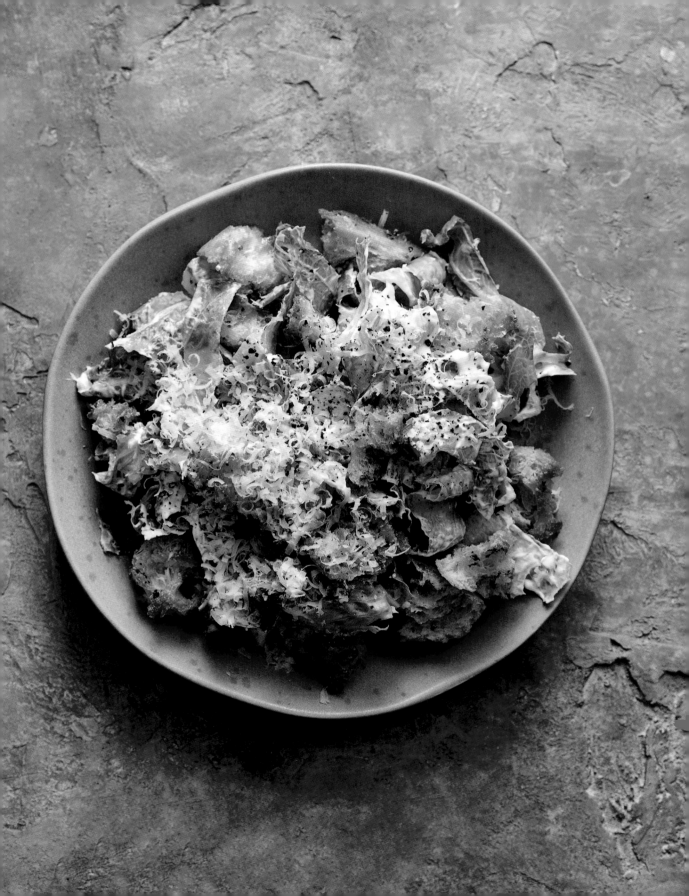

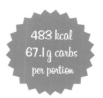

483 kcal
67.1g carbs
per portion

MEXICAN FAUX-PASTRY WRAPS

Puff pastry is a great idea for food on the go, but it's high in calories and fat. So, I came up with a way to fake it: slices of bread! Just squash them down with your fingers or a rolling pin, and you have the perfect substitute. Here, I have stuffed my wraps with spiced butternut squash as well as black beans to keep you full for longer. Top tip: keep the filling quite dry to avoid your wraps going soggy.

To make 1 portion (2 wraps)

¼ butternut squash, chopped into 1cm cubes

1 tsp ground cumin

1 tsp smoked paprika

2 spring onions, sliced

¼ tin of black beans (100g), drained

2 slices of bread

1 egg, beaten (optional)

Sprinkle of poppy seeds

Oil (any)

Salt and pepper

To cook

Preheat your oven to 180°C/gas mark 4 and line a baking tray.

Scatter the butternut squash on to another baking tray and drizzle over a splash of olive oil, then scatter over the cumin and paprika, salt and pepper. Roast for about 25 minutes, then slightly squash the butternut squash cubes with the back of a fork to create a lumpy, textured mash. Add the spring onions and black beans, then allow the mixture to cool a bit.

Meanwhile, take the slices of bread and squash them down using your fingers or a rolling pin. Spoon the filling diagonally across the slices. Fold the left and right sides over the filling (secure with a toothpick, if needed), then brush with the beaten egg (if using) and sprinkle with the poppy seeds. Lay the wraps on the prepared baking tray and cook for about 20 minutes, or until they are golden brown.

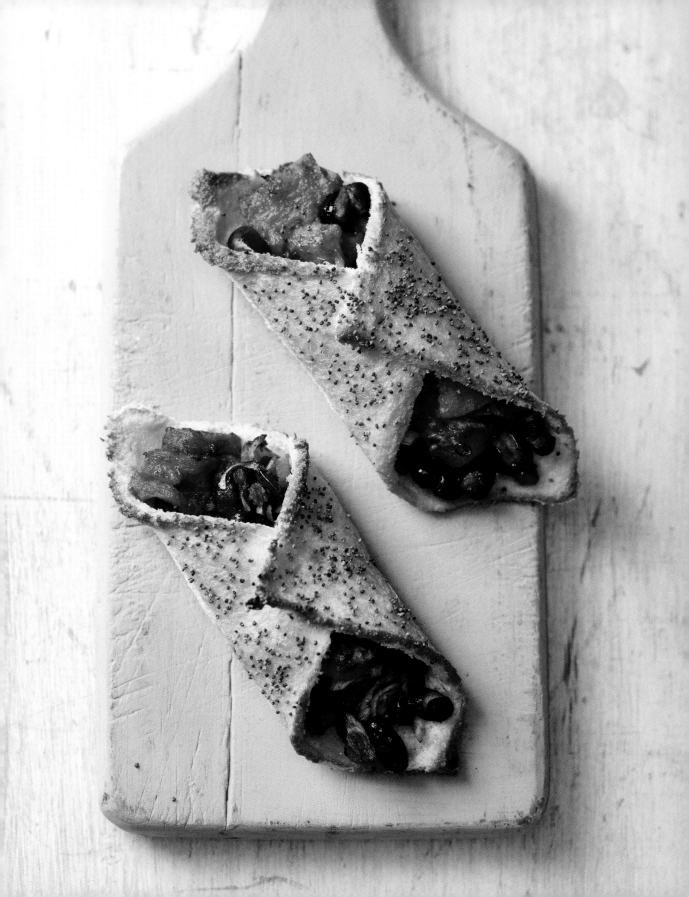

FROZEN PRAWN PHO

255 kcal
39.7g carbs
per portion

Easy, quick and delicious. I always have a bag of prawns in the freezer and noodles in the cupboard, so at a moment's notice, I can avoid an unplanned takeaway and get something equally delicious but far healthier. Prawns are a great source of protein and, with the noodles, this is a plate of food that will keep you satisfied for longer.

To make 1 portion

400ml water

½ stock cube (any flavour, but my favourite is chicken)

Handful of frozen prawns

Sheet of dried rice noodles

½ pak choi (or any green veg)

Big splash of soy sauce

1 tsp crispy chilli in oil

Small handful of chopped coriander (optional)

To cook

Bring the water to the boil in a saucepan. Crumble in the stock cube and stir to dissolve, then add the prawns, noodles and pak choi and simmer for a few minutes until the noodles are soft. Pour the broth into a bowl and add a big splash of soy sauce and the chilli. Garnish with chopped coriander, if using, then serve.

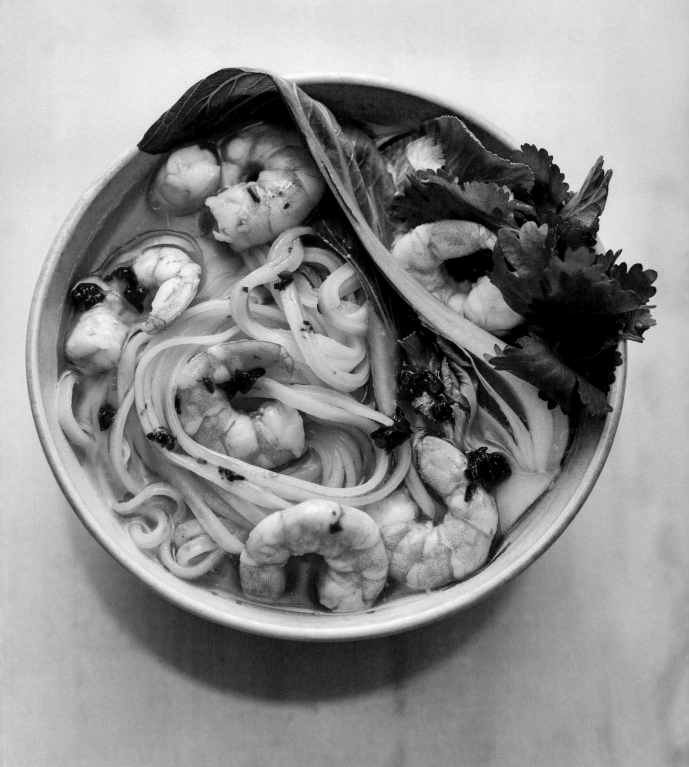

366 kcal
44.2g carbs
per portion

EGG KRAPOW

I thought I might have gone too far here by using egg instead of minced pork, but this actually works and it tastes fantastic. Eggs are so good for you. They're high in protein and healthy fats, making them a great choice for this dish because you'll feel fuller for longer. You're supposed to use Thai basil, but don't worry if you only have normal basil – it'll be okay.

To make 1 portion

¼ mug of rice

½ mug of water

A few green beans, halved

1 garlic clove, grated

2 eggs

A few slices of red chilli

A few basil leaves (Thai basil, if you have it)

Splash of soy sauce

Oil (any)

Salt and pepper

To cook

Put the rice, water and beans into a saucepan with a pinch of salt and cook over a medium heat with the lid on for about 10 minutes, until all the water has been absorbed and the rice is cooked. Remove the beans and set aside.

Fry the garlic in a splash of oil in a frying pan over a medium heat for about 30 seconds, then crack the eggs into the pan. Cook them for a few minutes until they're almost cooked through, then stir to break them up. Next add the soy sauce, chilli, basil and cooked green beans. Season and stir everything together for another minute, then serve with the rice.

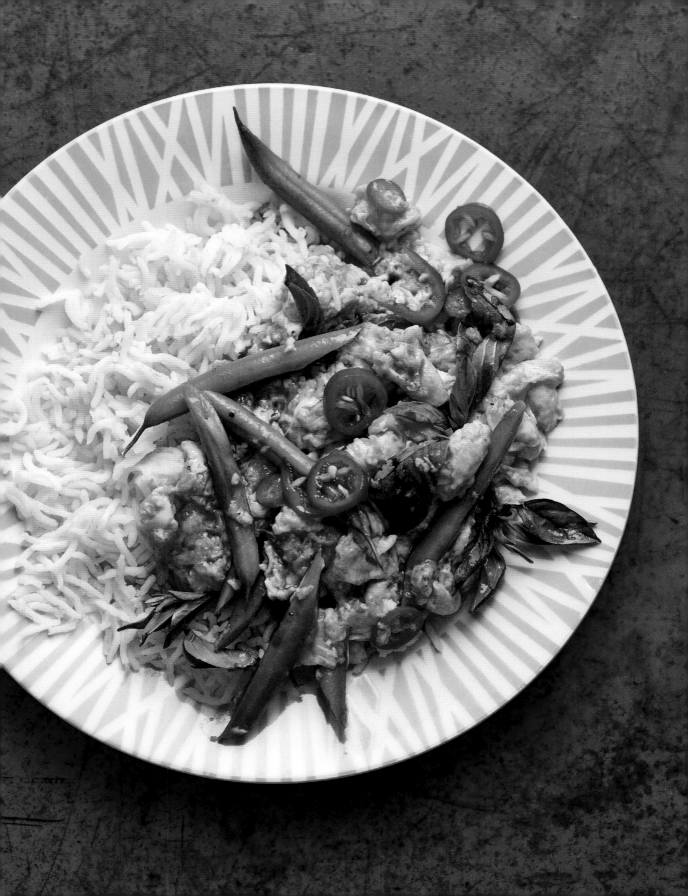

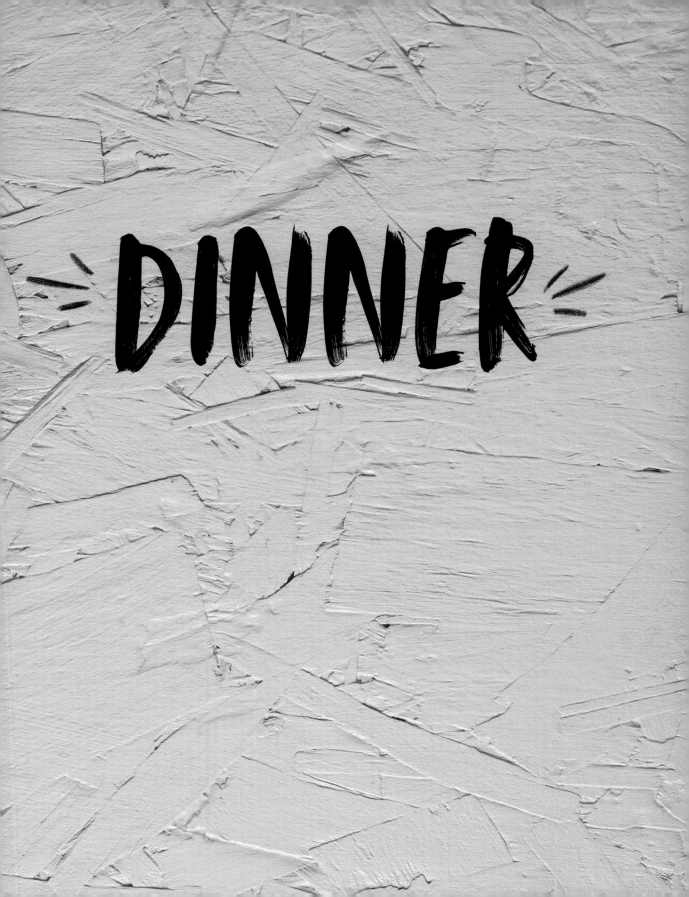

449 kcal
52.6g carbs
per portion

CAULI BURGERS

Another great way to substitute meat with vegetables. Get a bit of colour on these burgers to unlock the next level of flavour. This is the secret with cauliflower, and why I never boil it: when it caramelises, it gets super tasty.

To make 1 burger

¼ cauliflower, broken into florets

Small handful of breadcrumbs

1 egg, beaten

Burger bun

A few slices of tomato

A few slices of red onion

A few lettuce leaves

1 tsp mayonnaise

1 tsp ketchup

Oil (any)

Salt and pepper

To cook

Preheat your oven to 180°C/gas mark 4.

Place the cauliflower florets on a baking sheet, drizzle with oil and season with salt and pepper. Roast for about 25 minutes until softened and cooked through.

In a bowl, roughly mash the cauliflower with the back of a fork, add the breadcrumbs, then mix in the egg bit by bit until you can shape the mixture with your hands. Add a little more salt and pepper. Shape into a burger patty, then cook in a hot frying pan in a splash of oil over a medium heat for about 6 minutes on each side, or until cooked through and golden brown.

Build the burger in the bun to your liking, layering up tomato, red onion and lettuce, and a mixture of mayo and ketchup.

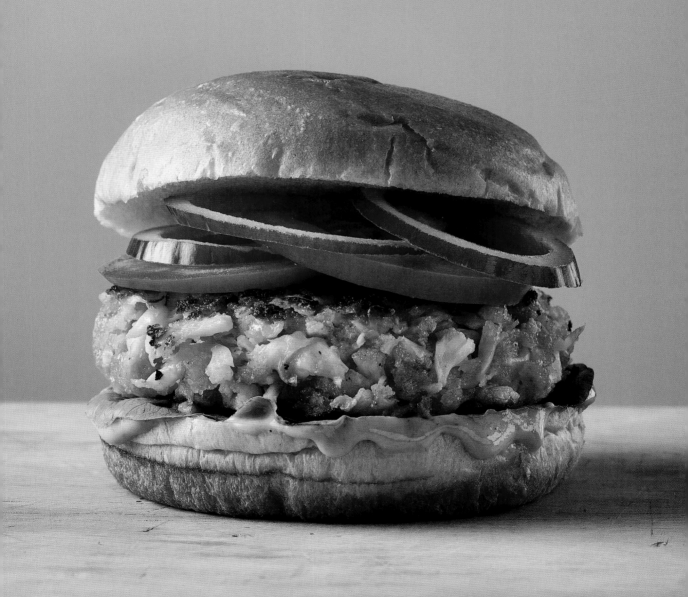

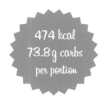

474 kcal
73.8g carbs
per portion

BACON BOLOGNESE

Want to cut down on the amount of meat in your bolognese? Then let bacon do all the hard work for you. Even a small amount of bacon will give the dish that meaty, smoky flavour you crave. If you let those bacon bits stick to the pan and caramelise, you can get an even deeper flavour.

To make 1 portion

75g any pasta

Handful of chopped smoky bacon or lardons

½ onion, sliced

1 carrot, diced

½ tin of chopped tomatoes (200g)

Olive oil

Salt and pepper

To cook

Cook the pasta in a pan of salted boiling water as per the instructions on the packet, then drain, reserving a mugful of the cooking water.

Meanwhile, pan-fry the bacon in a splash of olive oil over a medium heat for about 5–10 minutes until golden brown, adding the onion and carrot halfway through. Be sure to scrape off any sticky bits from the bottom of the pan. Then add the tomatoes, simmer for 10 minutes, adding a splash of the pasta cooking water if needed, then mix in the cooked pasta and serve.

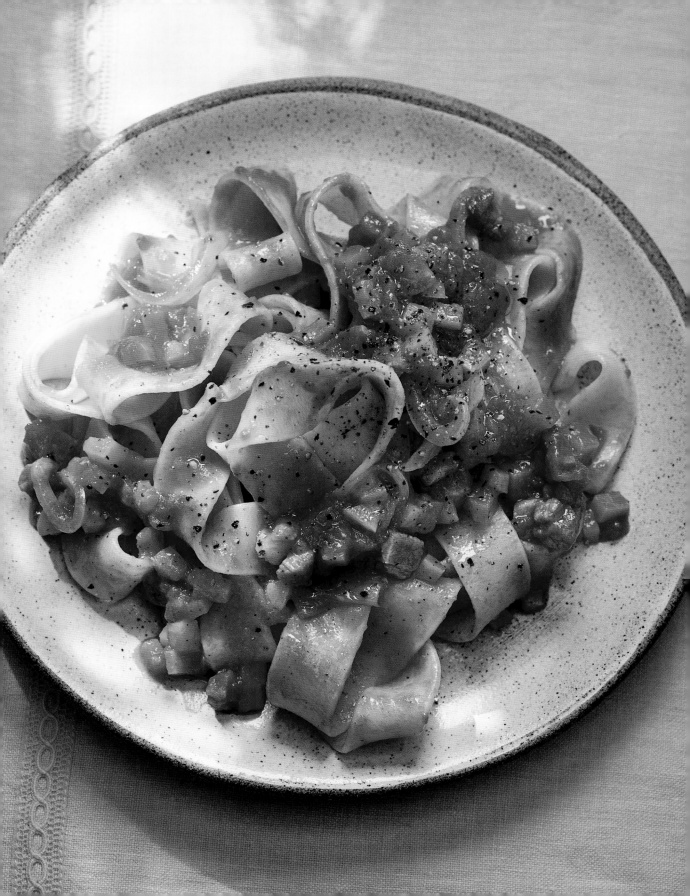

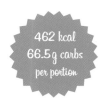

462 kcal
66.5 g carbs
per portion

BOMBAY POTATO FISH CAKES

This is a fun twist on my no-fuss fish cakes from one of my previous books. This time, we're taking the flavour up a level by using Bombay potatoes, and then going even further by using crushed poppadoms instead of breadcrumbs. But regular breadcrumbs are totally fine too, and you're more likely to have some bread at home. I'd hate to think you didn't make this dish because you didn't have any poppadoms.

To make 1 portion (3 fishcakes)

2 potatoes, cut into chunks

1 frozen (or fresh) skinned fish fillet (any fish)

Small handful of frozen peas

1 tsp curry powder

1 crushed poppadom (or a handful of breadcrumbs)

Handful of salad leaves

Lemon wedge

Oil (any)

Salt and pepper

To cook

Cook the potatoes in a pan of salted boiling water for about 15 minutes, or until cooked through, adding the fish and peas for the last few minutes. Drain in a colander and allow to steam-dry for a few minutes before tipping into a bowl and roughly crushing with the back of a fork. Mix in the curry powder, season, then shape into three patties. Scatter the crushed poppadom or breadcrumbs on to a plate and press both sides of each patty into them to coat. Pan-fry the fish cakes in a splash of oil over a medium heat, then serve with salad leaves and a lemon wedge for squeezing over.

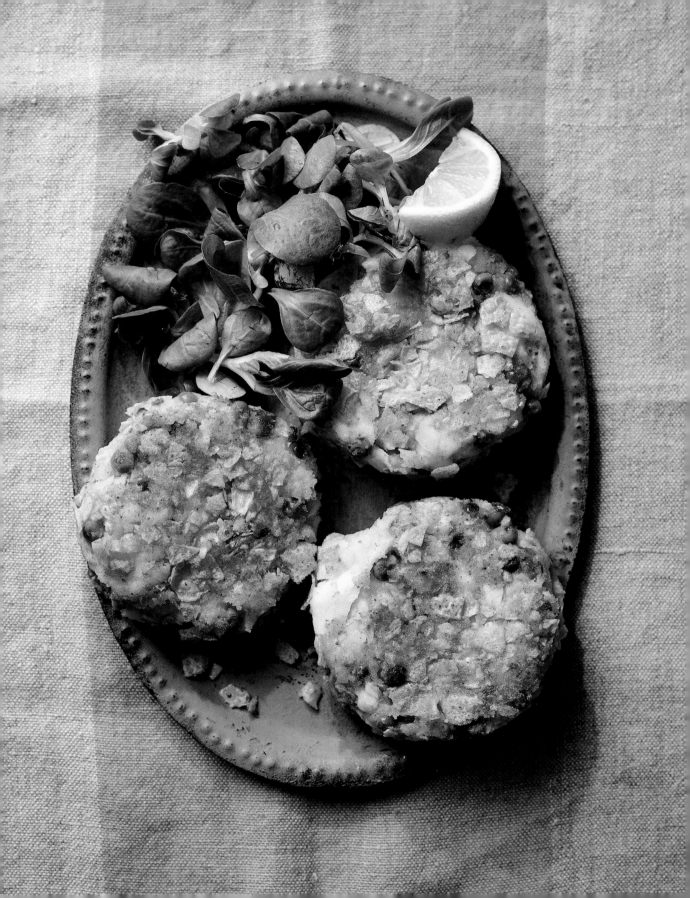

COCONUT CURRY

If you want to get some extra veg into your diet without noticing, just hide it in this creamy curry. I had some pak choi left over from my Frozen Prawn Pho recipe (page 94), plus some mini corn from one of those selection packs, so in they went! The key is to add the veg that takes longest to cook (the butternut squash) first and the veg that cooks fastest (the pak choi) last.

To make 1 portion

2 garlic cloves

A small piece of fresh root ginger

1 tbsp tomato purée

1 tsp curry powder

A few slices of red chilli

A few cubes of butternut squash

½ onion, sliced

2–3 mini sweetcorn, halved lengthways

½ tin of coconut milk (200ml)

½ pak choi, leaves separated

Small handful of chopped coriander (optional)

Oil (any)

Salt and pepper

To cook

Using your finest grater, grate the garlic and ginger into a small bowl, then add the tomato purée and curry powder, along with a splash of oil. Mix to create a paste.

Spoon the paste into a frying pan and add the chilli, butternut squash, onion, sweetcorn and a pinch of salt and pepper. Pan-fry over a medium heat, stirring frequently, for about 10 minutes.

Next, add the coconut milk, plus a splash of water, and simmer for about 10 minutes until the butternut squash is cooked (adding more water if needed). For the final couple of minutes, add the pak choi, then season to taste and serve with a sprinkle of coriander, if using.

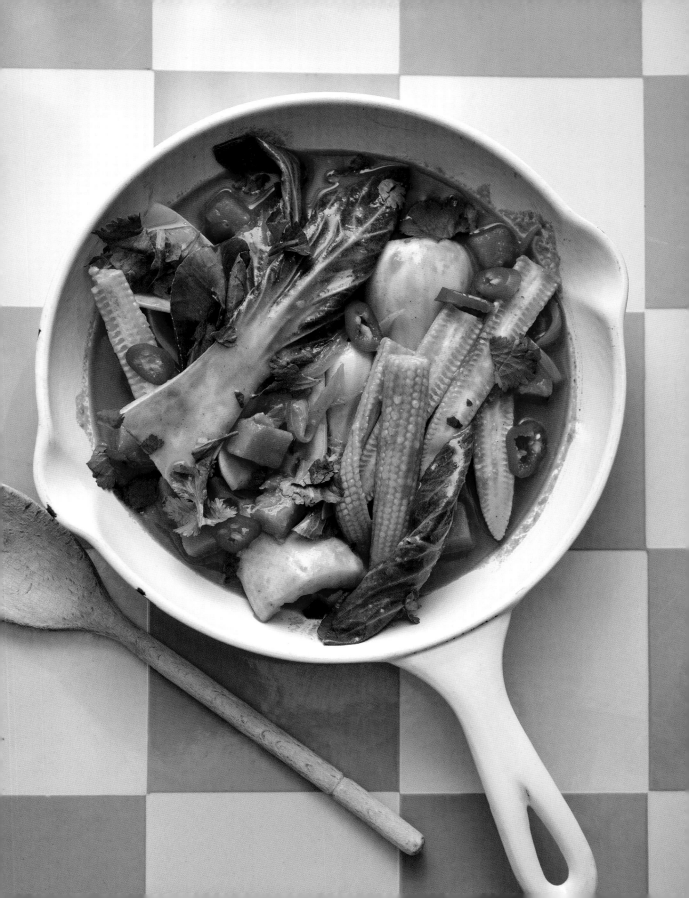

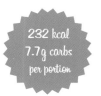

CANNELLINI BEAN PUTTANESCA

Here's a nice way to substitute pasta with some lovely high-fibre and high-protein cannellini beans, while still getting all those familiar puttanesca flavours from the garlic, capers and tomatoes.

To make 1 portion

1 garlic clove, sliced

Pinch of dried chilli flakes

1 tsp capers, plus a splash of the brine

½ tin of chopped tomatoes (200g)

½ tin of cannellini beans (200g), drained

Small handful of pitted black olives, halved

Sprinkle of chopped parsley, to garnish (optional)

Oil (any)

Salt and pepper

To cook

Pan-fry the garlic and chilli flakes in a splash of oil over a medium heat for a minute or so. Add the capers, and a splash of the brine, along with the chopped tomatoes, cannellini beans and olives. Season with salt and pepper, then simmer for 10–15 minutes, adding a splash of water if required. Garnish with parsley, if using, then serve.

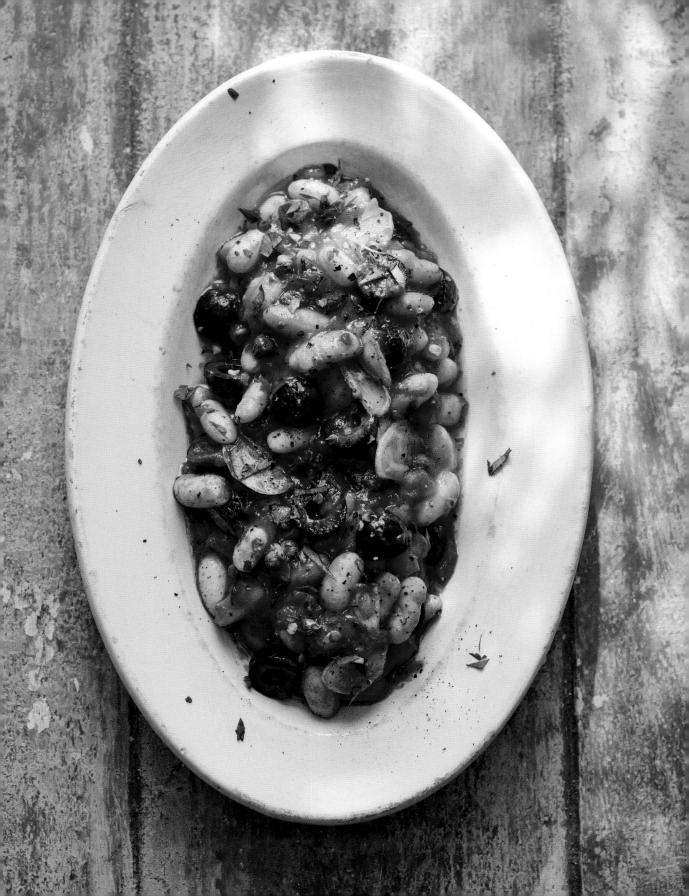

CHICKEN ROMESCO

This one is packed with flavour and even uses veg as the sauce. Substituting white rice for brown is also an easy swap that will help you hit your daily fibre target without you even noticing.

To make 1 portion

1 skinless chicken thigh

½ red pepper, seeded

2 garlic cloves, peeled but left whole

1 tomato

½ tsp smoked paprika

¼ mug of brown rice

½ mug of water

Oil (any)

Salt and pepper

To cook

Preheat your oven to 180°C/gas mark 4.

Chuck the chicken, red pepper, garlic and tomato into a roasting tin. Drizzle with oil and season with salt, pepper and the paprika. Roast for about 20 minutes until the chicken is cooked.

Meanwhile, put the rice and water into a saucepan with a pinch of salt and cook, covered, over a medium heat for about 10 minutes, until all the water has been absorbed and the rice is cooked.

Remove the chicken from the roasting tin and pour everything else into a blender, including all the juices. Blend until smooth (adding a splash of water if it is too thick), then serve the sauce with the chicken and rice.

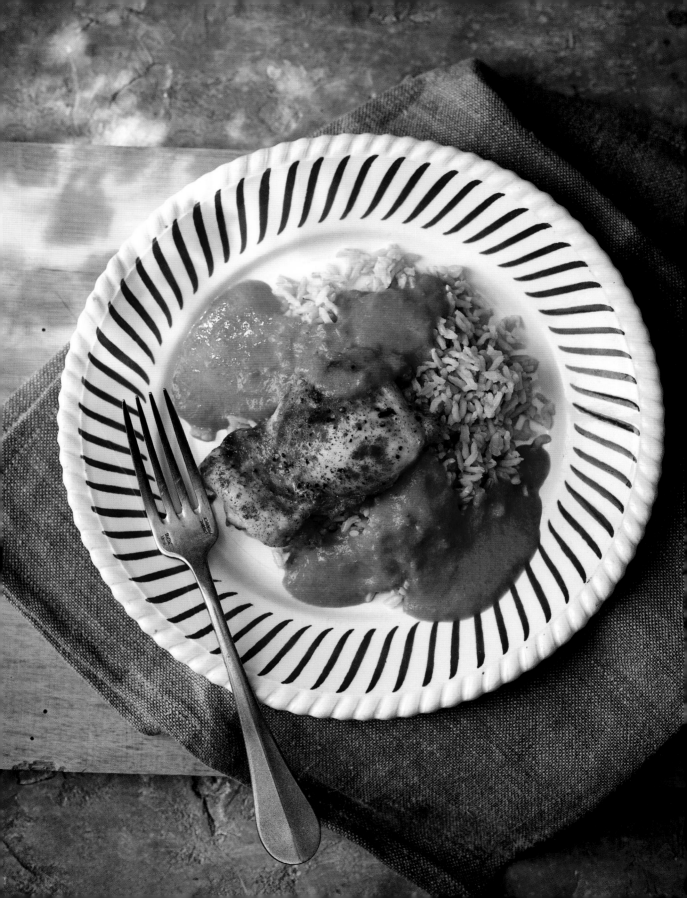

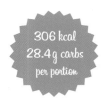

306 kcal
28.4g carbs
per portion

SUN-DRIED TOMATO PESTO GNOCCHI

Sun-dried tomatoes are one of the most powerfully flavoured ingredients you can buy. So, they are perfect for this punchy pesto, where a little goes a long way.

To make 1 portion

Handful of gnocchi

Large handful of rocket, plus extra for garnish

5–6 sun-dried tomatoes

Small handful of pine nuts, plus extra for garnish

1 garlic clove

Olive oil

Salt and pepper

To cook

Toast the gnocchi in a dry frying pan over a medium heat for about 10 minutes until they start to colour nicely.

Meanwhile, add the rocket, sun-dried tomatoes, pine nuts and garlic to a blender or food processor, along with a big glug of olive oil and the same amount of water. Season with salt and pepper, then blitz into a sauce, adding more water if it is too thick.

Tip the gnocchi on to a plate, spoon over the pesto, and garnish with a few rocket leaves and some pine nuts.

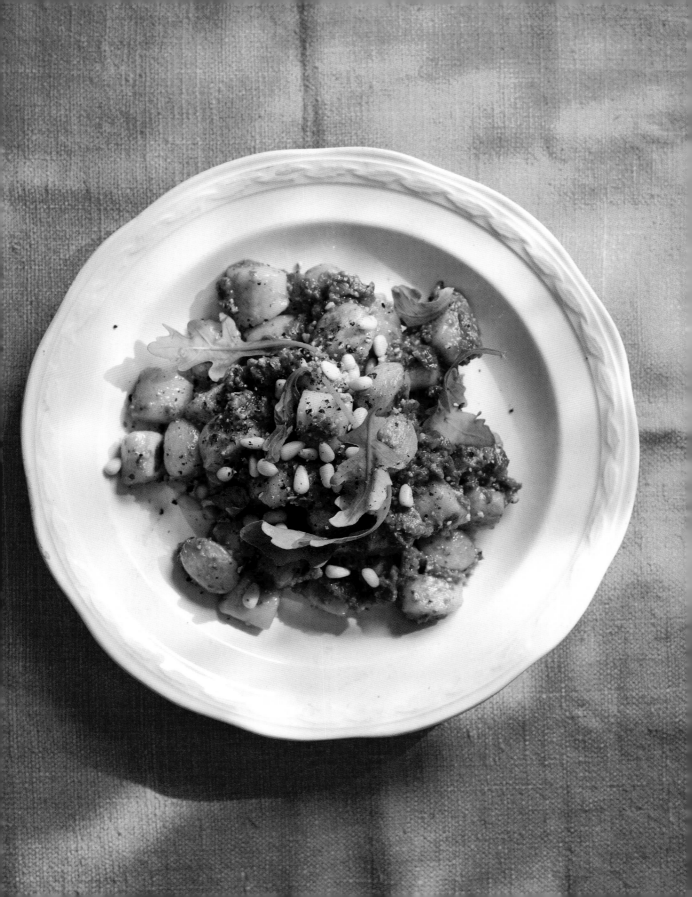

387 kcal
47.8g carbs
per portion

CHICKEN & ROOT VEG HOTPOT

Nice and filling, this is packed with veg and chicken and topped with potatoes – everything you need for cosy comfort food. A lovely balanced meal made with minimal effort.

To make 1 portion

1 skinless chicken thigh

½ onion, sliced

1 carrot, roughly chopped

½ tsp plain flour

½ stock cube (any flavour)

½ mug of water

1 potato, sliced

Pinch of dried oregano

Oil (any)

Salt and pepper

To cook

Preheat your oven to 180°C/gas mark 4.

Season and pan-fry the chicken thigh in a splash of oil over a medium heat for about 5 minutes on each side, adding the onion and carrot halfway through. Stir in the flour and continue to cook for a further minute before crumbling in the stock cube and adding the water. Stir and simmer for a couple of minutes. Remove the chicken and shred using two forks, then transfer everything to a small ovenproof dish. The liquid needs to cover the chicken and veg, so add more water if needed. Top with the sliced potato, drizzle with olive oil and sprinkle over salt, pepper and oregano. Cook in the oven for about 30 minutes, or until the potato looks golden and delicious.

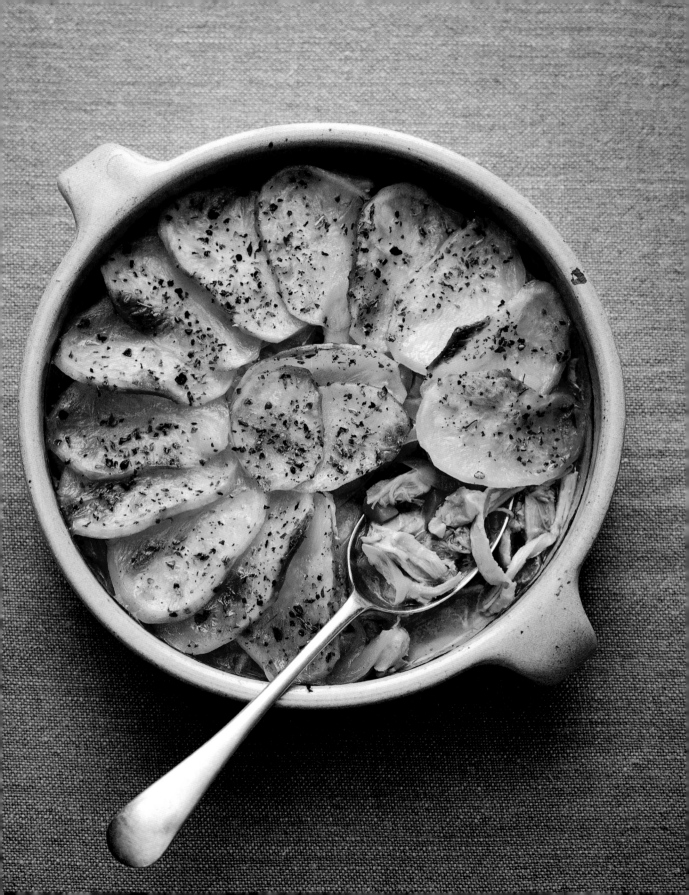

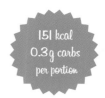

151 kcal
0.3g carbs
per portion

FLATTENED CHICKEN WITH CAPER JUS

The capers in this dish add a lively tang, making it a light and summery recipe. The key is to get lots of colour on the chicken, and the way to do this is to place something heavy on top. In Italy, they sometimes use a brick, but I like to use my casserole dish. My top tip here is to use a bit of baking parchment or tin foil as a barrier to prevent the raw chicken touching the bottom of the weight. You can serve this chicken with rice, couscous or potatoes, but if you want to keep it low carb, then salad is a great option, because all those flavours in the sauce will dress the salad beautifully for you.

To make 1 portion

2 chicken breast mini fillets

1 tbsp capers, plus a splash of the brine

Handful of chopped parsley (optional)

Oil (any)

Salt and pepper

To cook

Toss the chicken fillets in a splash of oil and season with a big pinch of salt and pepper. Arrange them in a frying pan, cover with a layer of baking parchment and place a heavy weight on top (I used a casserole dish). Pan-fry over a medium heat for about 5–7 minutes, or until nicely coloured on the bottom, then flip them over, discarding the baking parchment, and cook the other side for a similar amount of time with the weight on top until nicely coloured.

Remove the chicken from the pan and set aside. Add the capers and a splash of the brine to the pan. Stir to release all the caramelised bits from the base of the pan and create a sauce. Return the chicken to the pan to warm through, and add a sprinkle of parsley before serving.

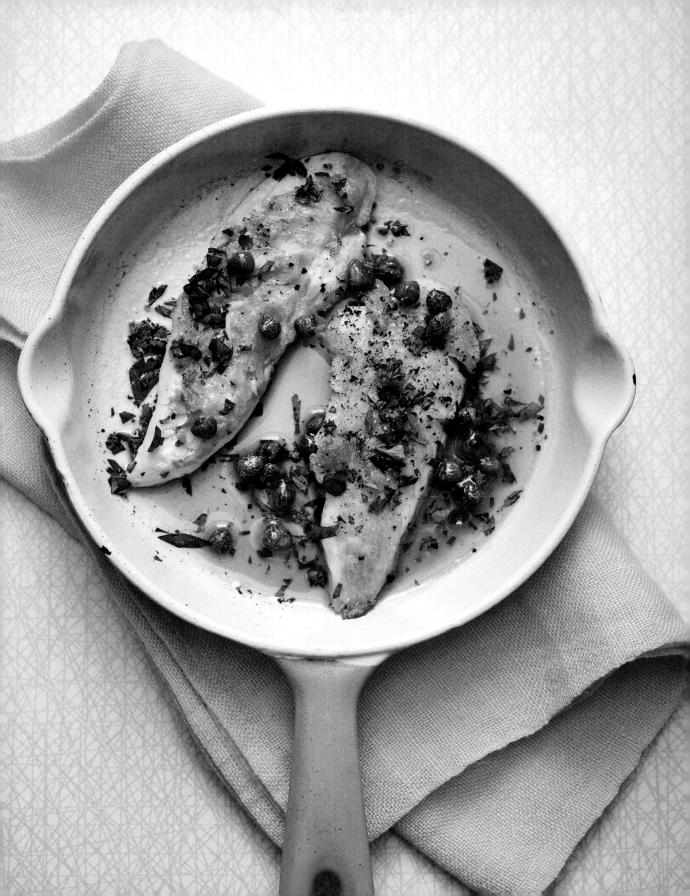

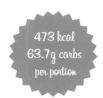

BROKEN SPAGHETTI

Lots of people have tried to cook their pasta in the same pot as the sauce, because technically it does make sense from a laziness perspective. But shaped pasta takes up too much room in a frying pan, and thin pasta is too long, so it can actually end up being more effort. So, I came up with the idea of watering down the sauce a bit, snapping the spaghetti into pieces and just chucking it all in. It's a sort of hybrid between spaghetti pomodoro and minestrone soup, but all you need to know is that it's quick, easy, delicious and healthy.

To make 1 portion

1 garlic clove, sliced

200g tomato passata or ½ tin of chopped tomatoes

75g spaghetti, roughly snapped into 5cm pieces

½ mug of water

Small handful of grated Parmesan

A few basil leaves

Olive oil

Salt and pepper

To cook

Pan-fry the garlic in a splash of oil over a medium heat for a minute before adding the tomato passata or chopped tomatoes and the broken spaghetti. Season, add the water, then simmer for about 10 minutes (adding more water if needed) until the pasta is cooked. Spoon into a bowl and finish with the Parmesan, basil, a pinch more pepper and a drizzle of olive oil.

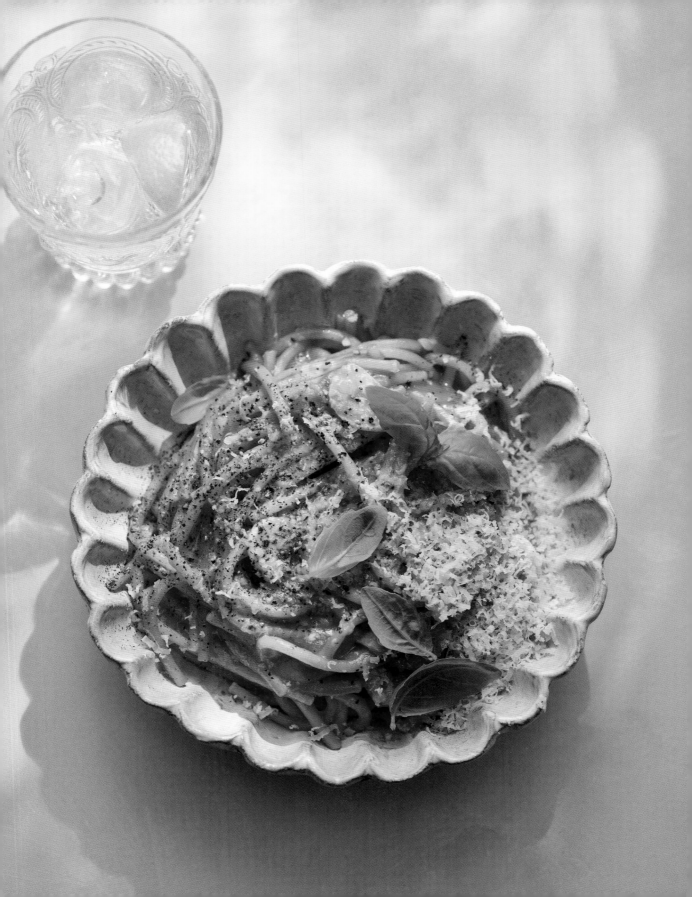

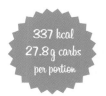

337 kcal
27.8g carbs
per portion

COURGETTE LASAGNE

A healthier, low-carb version of a classically heavy dish. Here, I have swapped out the pasta sheets for some lighter and more vibrant sliced courgettes. I've used whole tinned tomatoes to give each layer a bit of body, but it works equally well with chopped tinned tomatoes; the layers will just be slightly more compact.

To make 1 portion

½ onion, sliced

1 garlic clove, sliced

400g tin whole tomatoes

A few pinches of dried oregano

2 courgettes, sliced lengthways

Handful of grated Cheddar cheese

Oil (any)

Salt and pepper

To cook

Preheat your oven to 190°C/gas mark 5.

Pan-fry the onion in a splash of oil over a medium heat for about 5 minutes until softened. Add the garlic and cook for another minute or so, then add the tomatoes. Season with salt, pepper and a pinch of oregano, and simmer for about 10 minutes.

Assemble the lasagne in an ovenproof dish. Start with a layer of tomato, then some courgette slices, then some grated Cheddar. Top with a pinch more of oregano, then go back to the tomato. Repeat until the dish is full, then bake in the oven for about 15–20 minutes and serve.

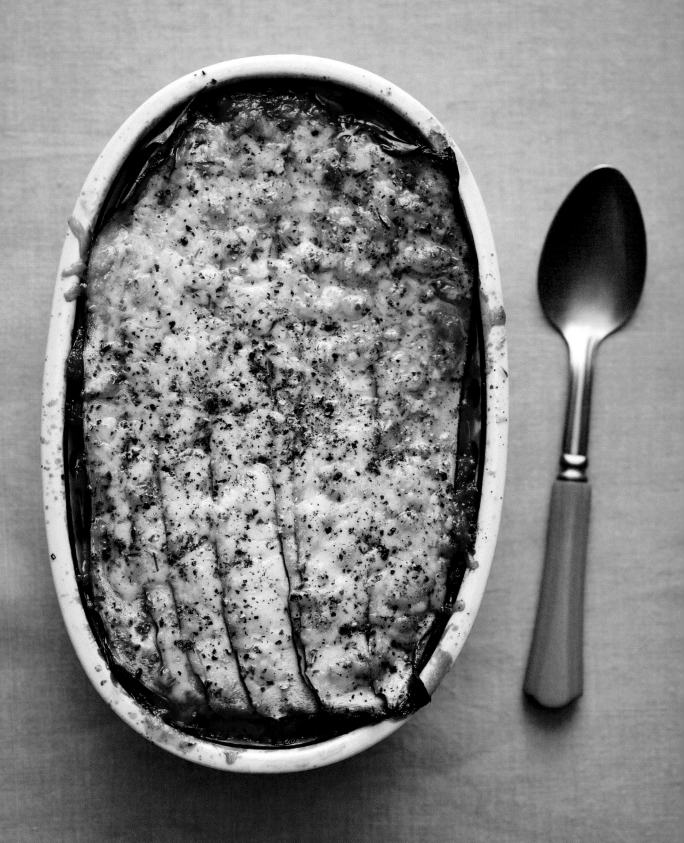

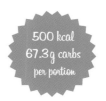

500 kcal
67.3g carbs
per portion

NO-BOIL PASTA BAKE

Easy-peasy dinner ideas are so important in order to avoid the dreaded takeaway. You need a few weapons in your arsenal that are guaranteed to hit the spot at a moment's notice – and this is one of them.

To make 1 portion

Big handful of pasta shells

½ red onion, diced

½ courgette, roughly diced

½ tin of chopped tomatoes (200g)

1 tsp dried oregano

1 mug of water

½ mozzarella ball, torn into chunks

Salt and pepper

To cook

Preheat your oven to 180°C/gas mark 4.

Grab an ovenproof dish and throw in the pasta, onion, courgette and chopped tomatoes. Sprinkle over the oregano and pour in the water. Season well, then stir and top with the chunks of mozzarella. Bake in the oven for about 30 minutes, or until the pasta is cooked and the cheese is bubbling. Serve.

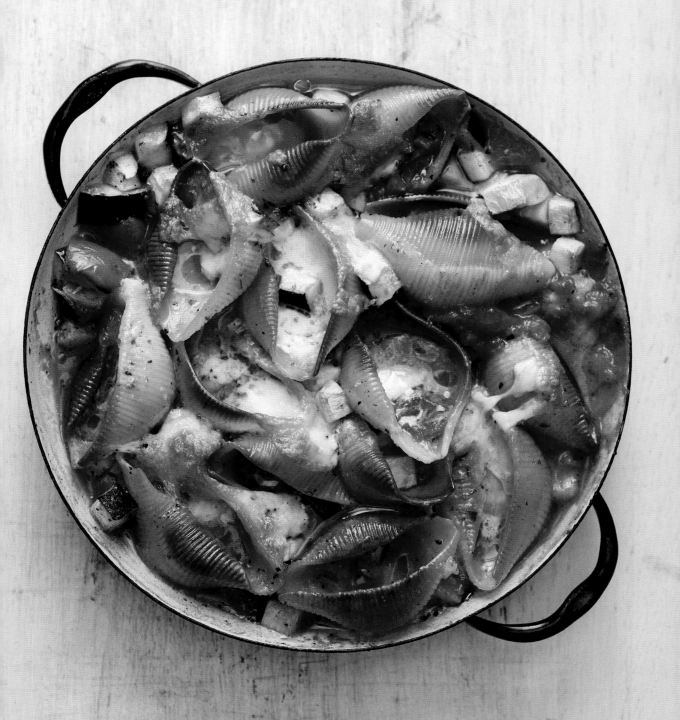

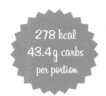

NO-CHEESE RISOTTO

If you take this usually rich dish in a lighter, fresher direction, then you can avoid the cheese. This is a summery, lemony risotto with a white wine base that perfectly complements the asparagus and prawns.

To make 1 portion

½ onion, diced

Handful of Arborio risotto rice

Splash of white wine

½ stock cube (any flavour)

500ml boiling water (approx.)

Juice and zest of ¼ lemon

Small handful of frozen king prawns

A few asparagus spears, roughly chopped

Oil (any)

Salt and pepper

To cook

Pan-fry the onion in a splash of oil over a medium heat for a few minutes until just before it starts to colour. Season, then add the risotto rice and toast in the pan for a couple of minutes before adding the wine. Cook for a further couple of minutes until the wine has almost evaporated. Crumble in the stock cube and add 100ml of the boiling water. Keep stirring and adding more water, 100ml at a time, until the rice is cooked and there is a nice amount of liquid in the pan. This should take around 15–20 minutes. Now add the lemon juice, prawns and asparagus. Mix everything together and, after a couple of minutes, remove from the heat. Grate over the lemon zest and add a splash more water if it is too sticky, then serve.

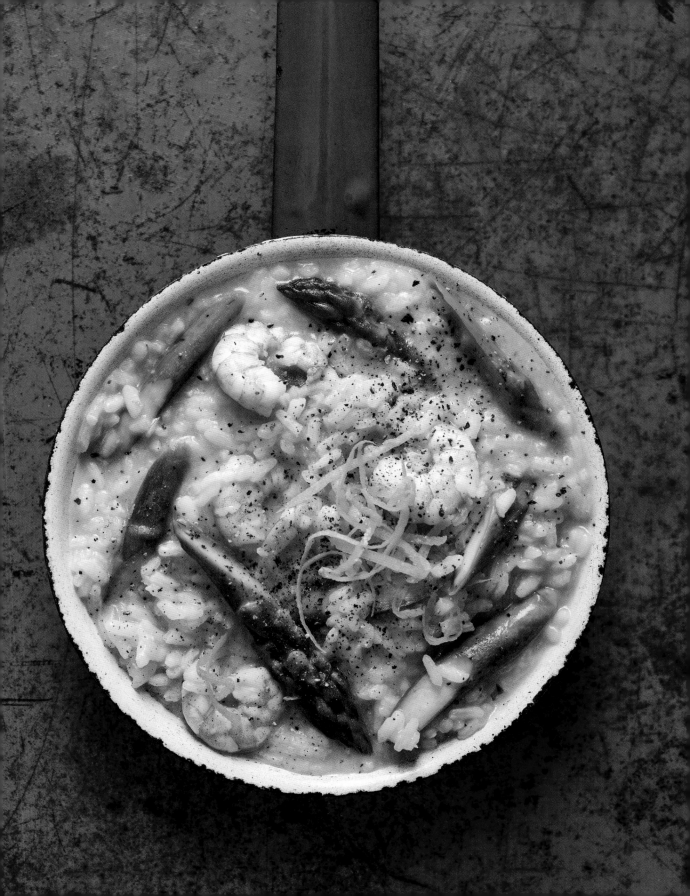

LENTIL CHILLI BOWL

Here is a hearty bowl of comfort food for you to enjoy. Lentils and beans are full of fibre and guaranteed to fill you up. They are also a great source of protein for vegetarians and vegans. Just swap out the crème fraîche and use a vegan stock cube and this can be a totally vegan dish.

To make 1 portion

½ onion, diced

½ tsp ground cumin

½ tsp smoked paprika

½ tin of chopped tomatoes (200g)

Handful of dried green lentils

½ vegetable stock cube

¼ tin of kidney beans (100g)

¼ mug of brown rice

½ mug of water

Dollop of crème fraîche

Small handful of chopped coriander (optional)

1 red chilli, seeded and sliced (optional)

Oil (any)

Salt and pepper

To cook

Pan-fry the onion in a splash of oil over a medium heat for about 5 minutes until softened. Add the cumin and paprika, and stir for a minute, then add the chopped tomatoes and lentils. Crumble in the stock cube and add a splash of water. Simmer for about 20 minutes, with the lid on, until the lentils are cooked, adding more water if needed. Season well and add the kidney beans for the last few minutes.

Meanwhile, put the rice and water into a saucepan with a pinch of salt and cook over a medium heat, covered, for about 10 minutes until all the water has been absorbed and the rice is cooked.

Serve the rice and chilli in a bowl with a dollop of crème fraîche, topped with some chopped coriander and chilli slices, if using.

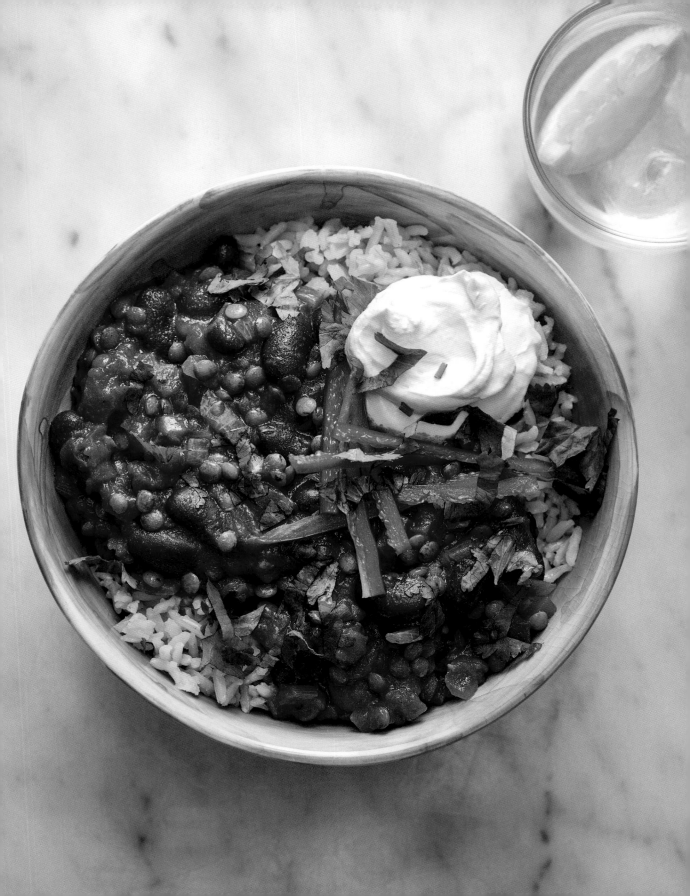

ROCKET PESTO LASAGNE SHEETS

I once went to a restaurant that used lasagne sheets in a dish and called them 'silk handkerchiefs'. They had crinkly edges, but I knew what was going on, they were just posh lasagne sheets! Anyway, I paid £12 for it, it looked cool and it was delicious. If you want this to be as close as possible to that restaurant version, then use fresh lasagne sheets, but if you want the vegan alternative then use dried sheets.

To make 1 portion

Large handful of rocket

Small handful of pine nuts

1 garlic clove

A few lasagne sheets (either fresh or dried)

Olive oil

Salt and pepper

To cook

Add the rocket, pine nuts and garlic to a blender or food processor, along with a big glug of olive oil and the same amount of water. Season with salt and pepper, then blitz into a sauce, adding more water if it is too thick.

Meanwhile, cook the pasta in a pan of salted boiling water as per the instructions on the packet, then drain.

Spoon the pesto over the pasta and scrunch it up a bit to get some height, then serve.

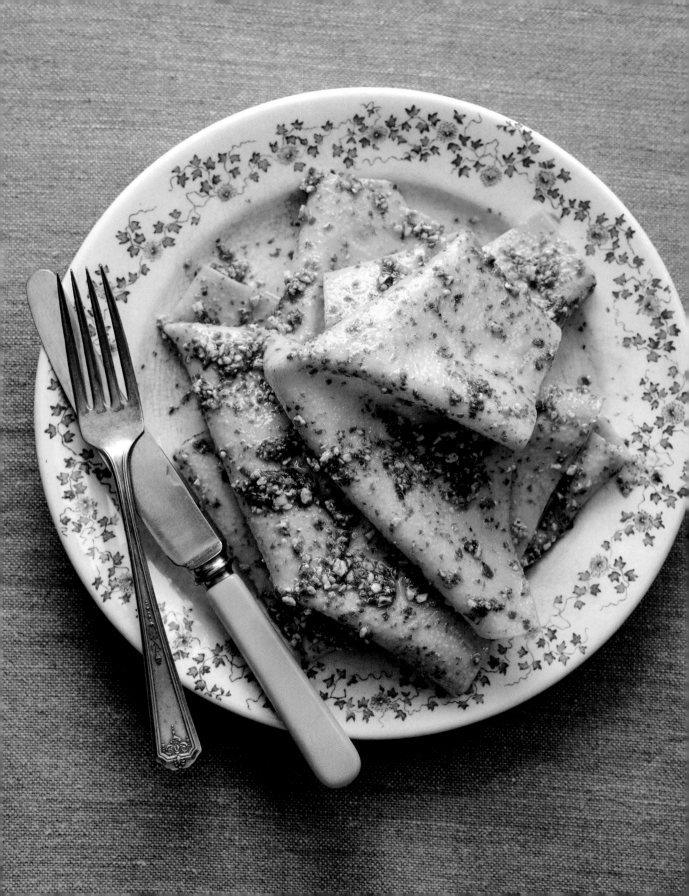

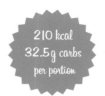

210 kcal
32.5g carbs
per portion

STICKY BLACK PEPPER NOODLES

The easiest way to get that fiery Szechuan flavour is to use pepper, just plain old pepper, the same one that you use every day, but lots of it. Udon noodles are low in fat, and broccoli increases the nutrient content as well as the fibre content.

To make 1 portion

½ pack of soft udon noodles (about 100g)

A few broccoli florets

1 garlic clove, sliced

A few slices of red chilli

½ tsp vegetable gravy granules

½ tsp tomato ketchup

Splash of soy sauce

Sesame oil

Salt and pepper

To cook

Cook the noodles in a pan of salted boiling water for 10 minutes, adding the broccoli halfway through, then drain, reserving a small mugful of the cooking water.

Meanwhile, pan-fry the garlic and ¼ teaspoon of black pepper in a splash of sesame oil over a medium heat for a couple of minutes, then add the chilli, gravy granules, tomato ketchup and soy sauce. Add the cooked noodles, broccoli and a splash of the reserved cooking water. Mix everything together and cook for a further couple of minutes until the sauce is reduced and sticky, then serve.

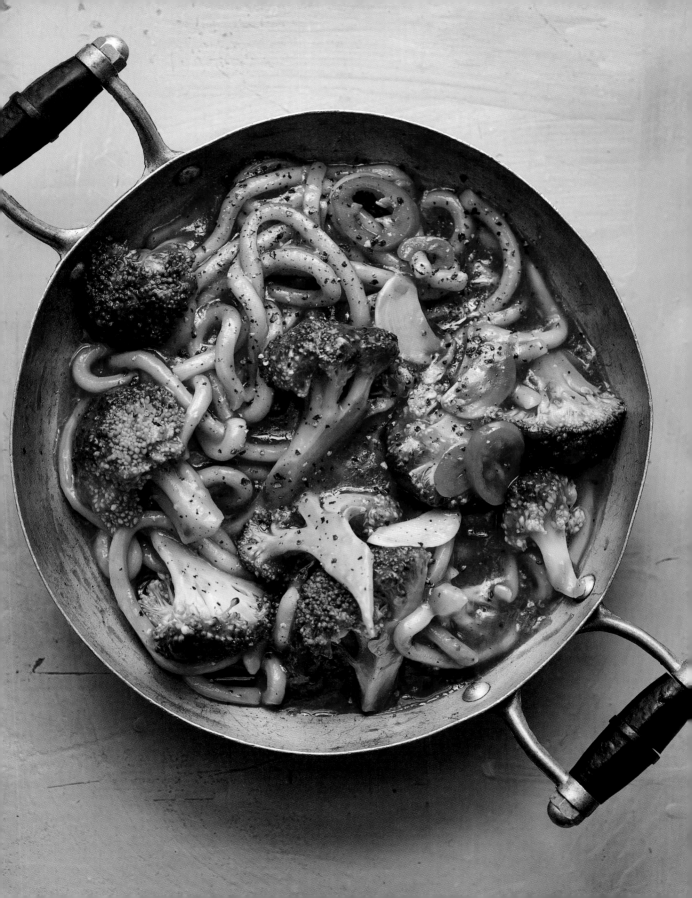

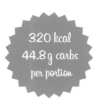

SUN-DRIED TOMATO & ASPARAGUS ORZO

This is a luxurious orzo that uses just a small amount of cream cheese to finish the dish and transform it into something very special, but without all the calories of a traditional cheese sauce.

To make 1 portion

½ onion, diced

A few sun-dried tomatoes, plus a splash of oil from the jar

Handful of orzo

½ mug of water

½ vegetable stock cube

A few asparagus spears, roughly chopped

1 tbsp cream cheese

Salt and pepper

To cook

Pan-fry the onion in a splash of oil from the sun-dried tomato jar over a medium heat for about 5 minutes. Once the onion is softened nicely, add the sun-dried tomatoes and orzo and stir together. Add the water, then crumble in the stock cube and season with a pinch each of salt and pepper. Simmer for about 10–15 minutes, stirring every so often, until the orzo is cooked, adding more water if needed.

Place the asparagus spears on top for the last few minutes, then stir through the cream cheese and serve.

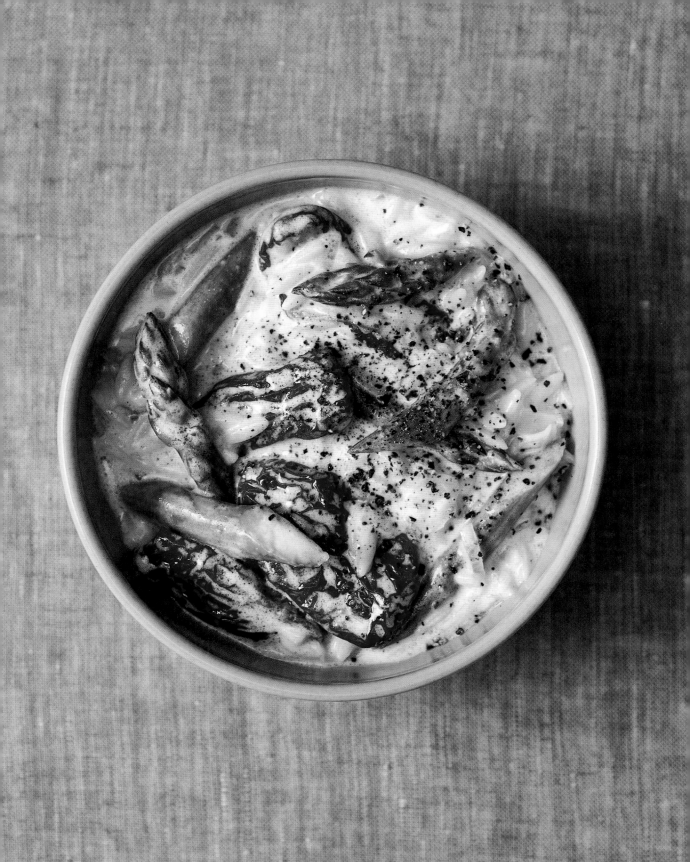

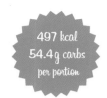

497 kcal
54.4g carbs
per portion

CHORIZO & CHICKPEA STEW

Just a little chorizo is all that is required here, because the paprika-infused oils will flavour this stew beautifully. This classic Spanish stew includes potatoes making it a complete meal in just one pan.

To make 1 portion

½ onion, sliced

A few slices of chorizo

1 potato, roughly diced

1 garlic clove, sliced

½ tin of chopped tomatoes (200g)

¼ tin of chickpeas (100g), plus ¼ of the liquid from the tin

½ chicken stock cube

Handful of frozen peas

Oil (any)

Salt and pepper

To cook

Pan-fry the onion, chorizo and potato in a splash of oil over a medium heat for about 5 minutes, then add the garlic and continue to cook for a couple more minutes. Next, add the chopped tomatoes, chickpeas and some of the liquid from the tin, then crumble in the stock cube. Simmer for about 10 minutes, or until the potato is cooked, then season to taste. Finally, add the peas and cook for a minute or so, then serve.

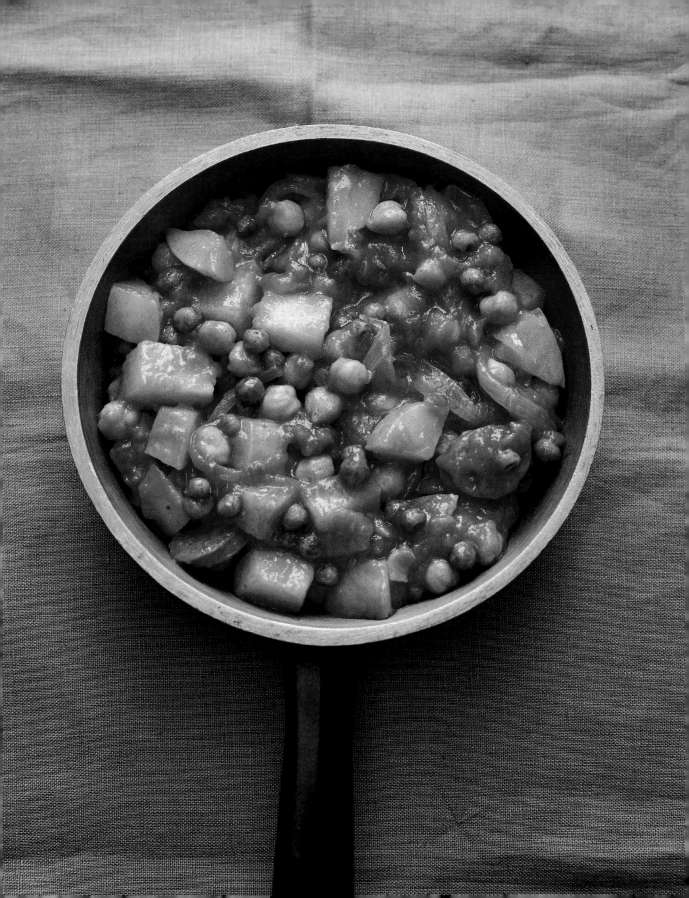

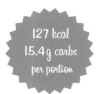

127 kcal
15.4g carbs
per portion

BEAN SPROUT NOODLES

Bean sprouts are a great low-carb substitute for noodles. They're basically just water, and therefore very low in calories, but they can still hold their own in this delicious stir-fried dish.

To make 1 portion

½ red onion, sliced

2 garlic cloves, sliced

Handful of green beans

½ carrot, cut into matchsticks

Handful of bean sprouts

1 tsp vegetable gravy granules

Pinch of dried chilli flakes

Splash of soy sauce

Sesame oil

Salt and pepper

To cook

Pan-fry the onions in a splash of sesame oil over a high heat for a couple of minutes, then add the garlic and green beans. After a couple more minutes, add the carrots, bean sprouts and gravy granules. After a few minutes, when everything is piping hot but the veg are still a bit crunchy, season, then finish with a splash of soy sauce and a pinch of chilli flakes.

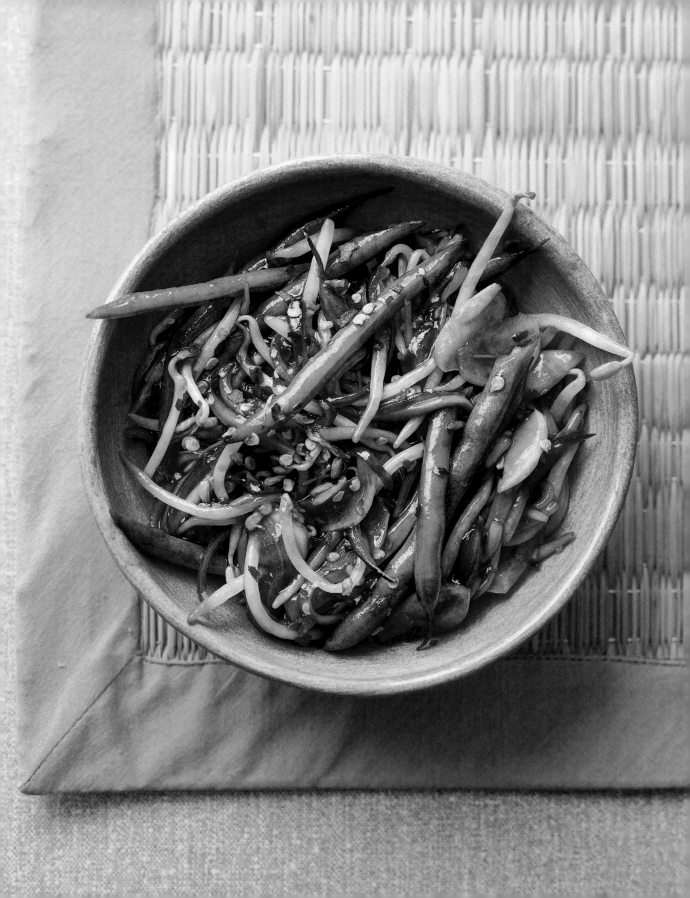

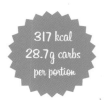

317 kcal
28.7g carbs
per portion

POLENTA & TINNED CHERRY TOMATOES

You can totally swap the tinned cherry tomatoes for normal chopped tomatoes, but if you're looking for a special treat that costs a tiny bit more, then you won't regret this. This is super fast and super simple – and far more delicious than you might expect.

To make 1 portion

½ onion, diced

2 garlic cloves, sliced

½ tin of cherry tomatoes (200g)

¼ mug of polenta

1¼ mugs of water

½ vegetable stock cube

Small handful of grated Cheddar cheese

Pinch of dried oregano

Olive oil

Salt and pepper

To cook

Pan-fry the onion in a splash of oil over a medium heat for about 5 minutes. Add the garlic and continue to cook for a couple of minutes before adding the tinned cherry tomatoes. Season, then leave to simmer for about 10 minutes.

Meanwhile, mix together the polenta and water in a saucepan, then crumble in the stock cube and add a pinch of salt and pepper. Bring to the boil, stirring. After about 10 minutes, once it is the consistency of porridge, remove from the heat and add the grated Cheddar.

Serve topped with the cherry tomatoes and a pinch of oregano.

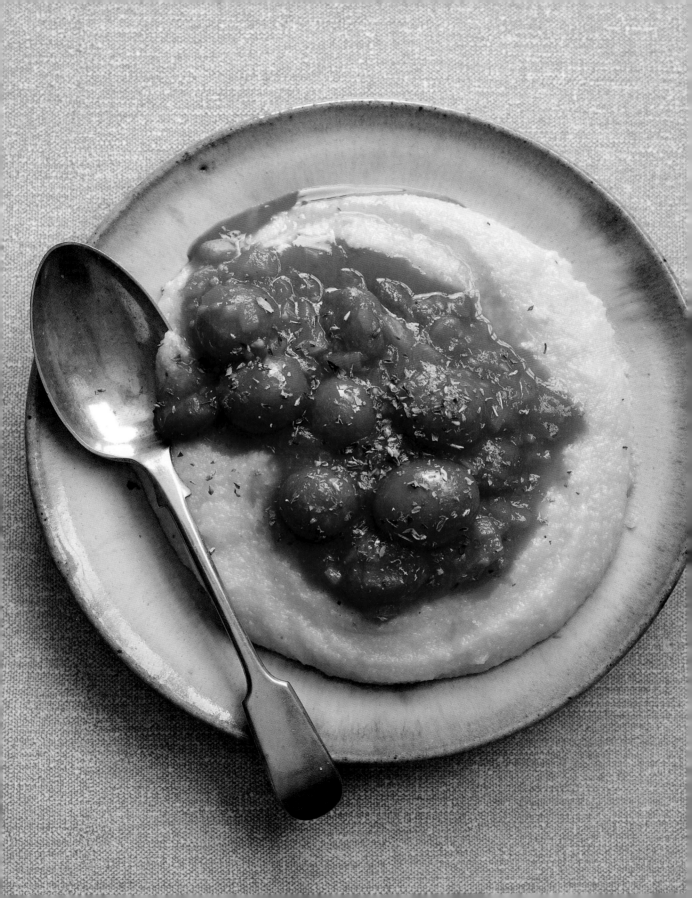

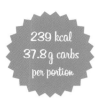

CAULIFLOWER GNOCCHI

This is for all those who crave gnocchi but are on a low-carb diet. Cauliflower gnocchi are easier to make than potato gnocchi, and more nutritious too. You can add whatever sauce you want, but I just like them pan-fried with sage and finished with a sprinkle of Parmesan.

To make 1 portion

½ cauliflower, broken into florets

2 tbsp plain flour, plus extra if needed

1 egg

A few sage leaves

Small handful of grated Parmesan

Oil (any)

Salt and pepper

To cook

Preheat your oven to 180°C/gas mark 4.

Scatter the cauliflower florets on to a baking sheet, then drizzle with olive oil and season with salt and pepper. Roast for about 25 minutes until cooked through. Transfer to a bowl, mash with a fork and mix in the flour and the egg. Very, very lightly knead the mixture on a worktop (don't press too hard, keep it fluffy) and shape into a sausage shape. If the mixture is too dry, add a splash of water; if it is too wet, add a sprinkle of flour.

Chop the sausage into 2cm sections. Pan-fry the gnocchi in a splash of oil over a medium–high heat for a few minutes, adding the sage leaves to the pan so they crisp up slightly. Serve sprinkled with grated Parmesan.

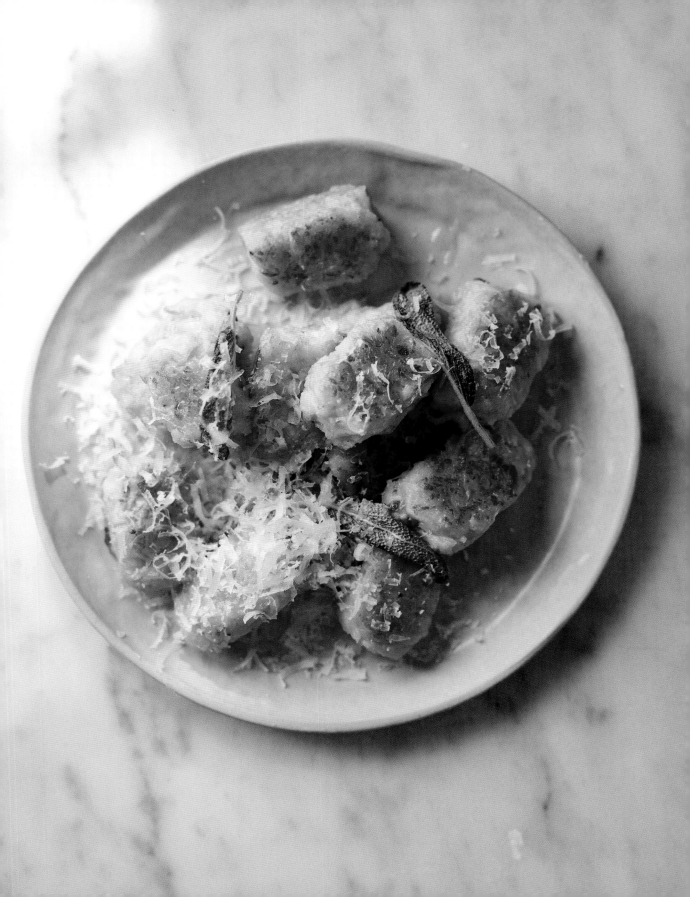

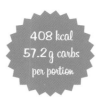

408 kcal
57.2 g carbs
per portion

PASTA ALLA SORRENTINA

This is just a posh way to say tomato pasta with melted cheese. You only need a small amount of mozzarella, because a little goes a long way! This is a nicely balanced meal, with protein, fat and carbs.

To make 1 portion

Handful of rigatoni pasta

1 garlic clove, sliced

Handful of cherry tomatoes, halved

¼ ball of mozzarella, roughly chopped

Small handful of chopped basil

Olive oil

Salt and pepper

To cook

Cook the pasta in a pan of salted boiling water as per the instructions on the packet, then drain, reserving a small mugful of the cooking water.

Meanwhile, pan-fry the garlic and cherry tomatoes in a splash of olive oil over a medium heat for about 5 minutes until the tomatoes are a bit squishy. Season, then add the cooked pasta, a splash of the pasta water, the mozzarella and the basil. Mix it all together and cook for a couple of minutes so the cheese melts, then serve.

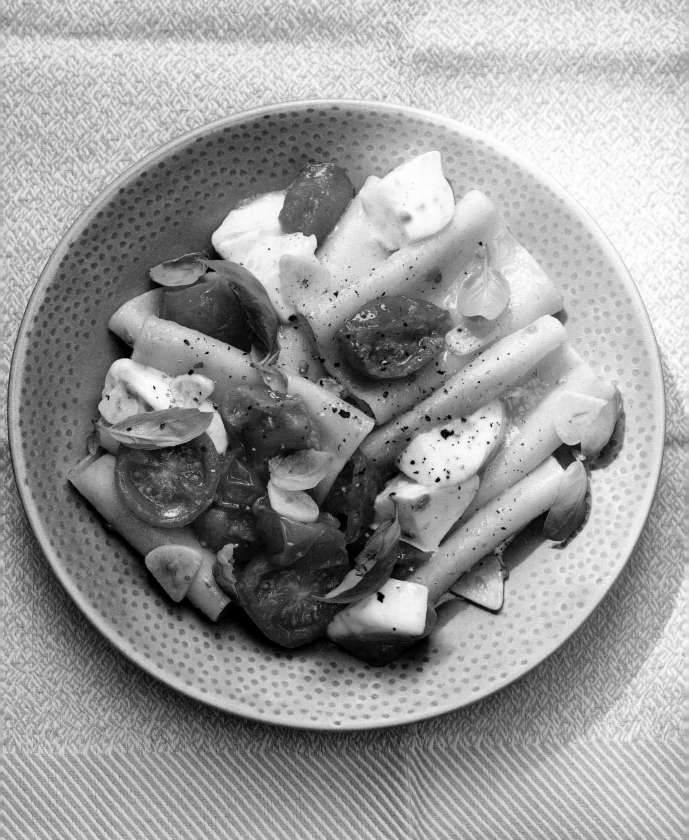

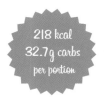

218 kcal
32.7g carbs
per portion

CHARRED GREEN BEAN STEW

I don't boil my beans anymore, I prefer to char them slightly, because it adds so much more flavour. Here, I have served them with a lovely protein-rich, low-calorie bean stew, flavoured with a pinch of smoky paprika.

To make 1 portion

½ onion, diced

1 garlic clove, sliced

½ tin of cannellini beans (200g), drained

½ tin of chopped tomatoes (200g)

Pinch of smoked paprika

½ vegetable stock cube

Handful of fine green beans

Oil (any)

Salt and pepper

To cook

Pan-fry the onion in a splash of oil over a medium heat for about 4 minutes, then add the garlic and continue to fry for a few more minutes. As soon as the garlic starts to colour, add the cannellini beans and chopped tomatoes. Season with salt, pepper and paprika, then crumble in the stock cube and simmer for about 15 minutes, adding a splash of water if it gets too dry.

Meanwhile, in a separate pan, season and fry the green beans in a splash of oil over a high heat for about 5 minutes until blistered and charred.

Serve the stew with the green beans piled on top.

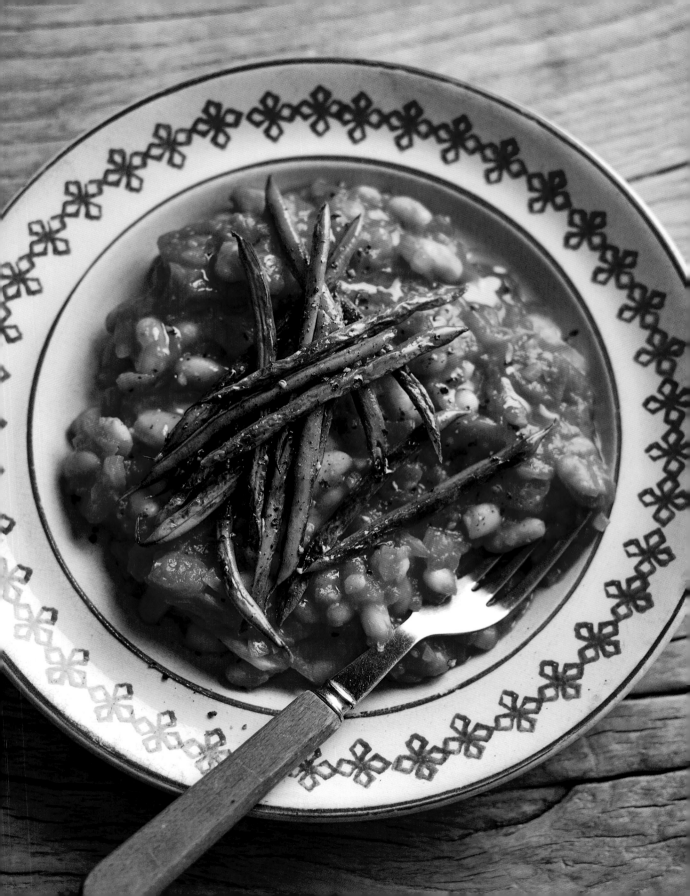

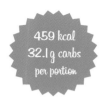

CASSOULET BLANCO

This is my version of a traditional cassoulet, using only one pan for a super-simple weekday meal. It's packed with protein and, as an added bonus, because of the beans, you don't really need any extra carbs. I love all-in-one meals.

To make 1 portion

1 chicken drumstick, skin-on

½ leek, sliced

1 garlic clove, sliced

¼ tsp plain flour

½ tin of cannellini beans (200g), plus ½ the liquid from the tin

100ml milk

½ chicken stock cube

Oil (any)

Salt and pepper

To cook

Preheat your oven to 180°C/gas mark 4.

In an ovenproof pan, season then fry the chicken in a splash of oil over a medium heat for about 5 minutes. Add the leek and continue to fry for another 5 minutes, then add the garlic and fry for 5 minutes more. Add the flour and stir it in until it disappears. Next, add the cannellini beans, plus the liquid, then pour in the milk and crumble in the stock cube. Season, then stir everything together. Bake in the oven for about 15 minutes until the chicken is totally cooked through and nicely coloured. Serve.

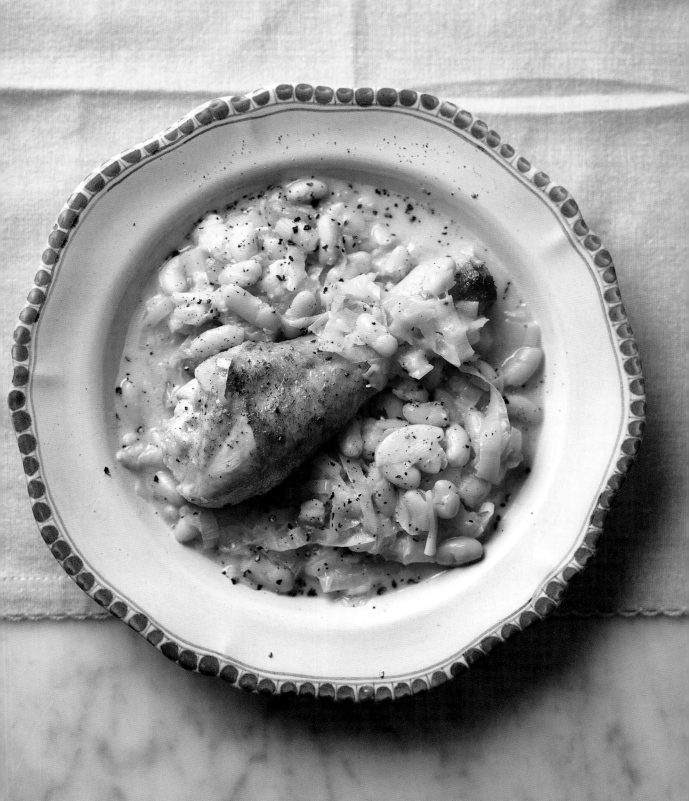

TOFU RENDANG

This is a well-balanced meal with protein-rich tofu. The key here is to get that scrambled-egg consistency, which most of the time you are battling to avoid, so this is probably the easiest recipe to try if you are unfamiliar with tofu.

To make 1 portion

¼ mug of rice

½ mug of water

¼ block of tofu (about 75g), crumbled

½ onion, sliced

1 garlic clove, sliced

1 tsp curry powder

½ tin of chopped tomatoes (200g)

1 egg

Small handful of chopped coriander

Oil (any)

Salt and pepper

To cook

Put the rice and water into a saucepan with a pinch of salt and cook over a medium heat with the lid on for about 7 minutes, until all the water has been absorbed and the rice is cooked.

Meanwhile, season and pan-fry the crumbled tofu and onion in a splash of oil over a medium heat for a few minutes until the onion starts to colour a little. Add the garlic and ½ teaspoon of the curry powder and continue to fry for a few more minutes. At this point, add the tomatoes and the remaining curry powder, season again, then simmer for about 15 minutes (adding a splash of water if it gets too dry).

When you are ready to serve, fry the egg in a separate pan in a splash of oil over a high heat until the white is set and crispy round the edges, but the yolk is still runny. Serve the tofu rendang on a bed of rice, topped with the egg and garnished with coriander.

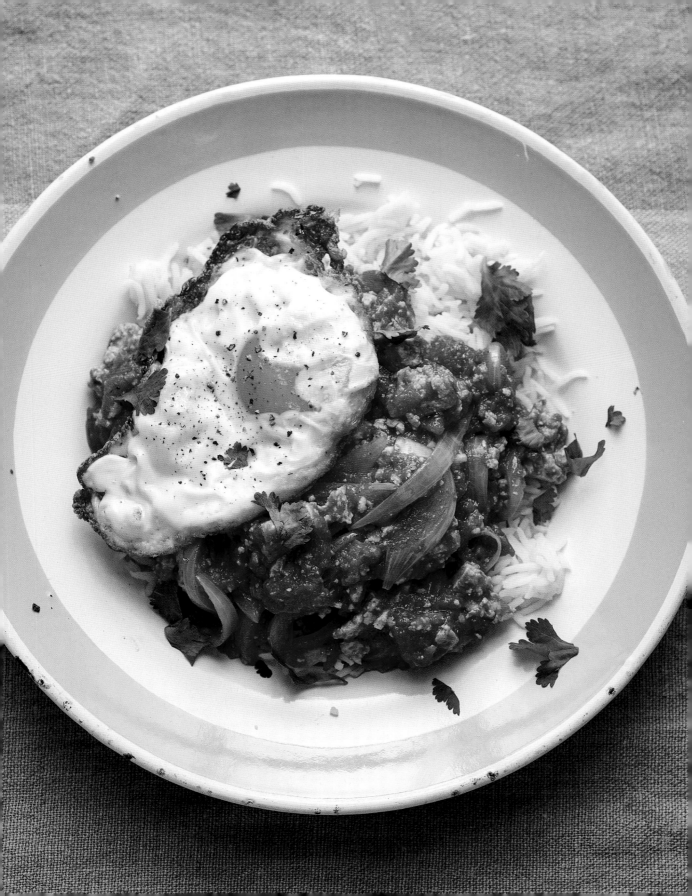

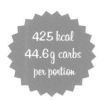

TRAY-BAKE FAJITAS

Minimal washing-up, maximum flavour: this is a delicious and nutritious meal that you can easily add to your existing routine. I like to cook my chicken thigh whole and slice it at the end to give neat, straight lines – not only does it look better, but this way you don't have to worry about raw chicken on your chopping board.

To make 1 fajita

1 skinless chicken thigh

Pinch of paprika

Pinch of ground cumin

½ onion, sliced

½ pepper, sliced

1 large tortilla wrap

Dollop of crème fraîche

Small handful of coriander (optional)

Oil (any)

Salt and pepper

To cook

Preheat your oven to 180°C/gas mark 4.

Place the chicken thigh in a baking tray. Mix a splash of oil with a pinch each of paprika, cumin, salt and pepper. Brush half the oil over the chicken thigh, then cook for about 10 minutes.

Next, add the veg to the tray and drizzle over the remaining oil mixture. Return to the oven for another 10–15 minutes.

Throw the wrap into the oven for the final minute of cooking to heat up. Remove everything from the oven, then slice the chicken.

Load up your wrap with chicken, roasted veg, crème fraîche and a sprinkle of coriander, if using. Roll up and serve.

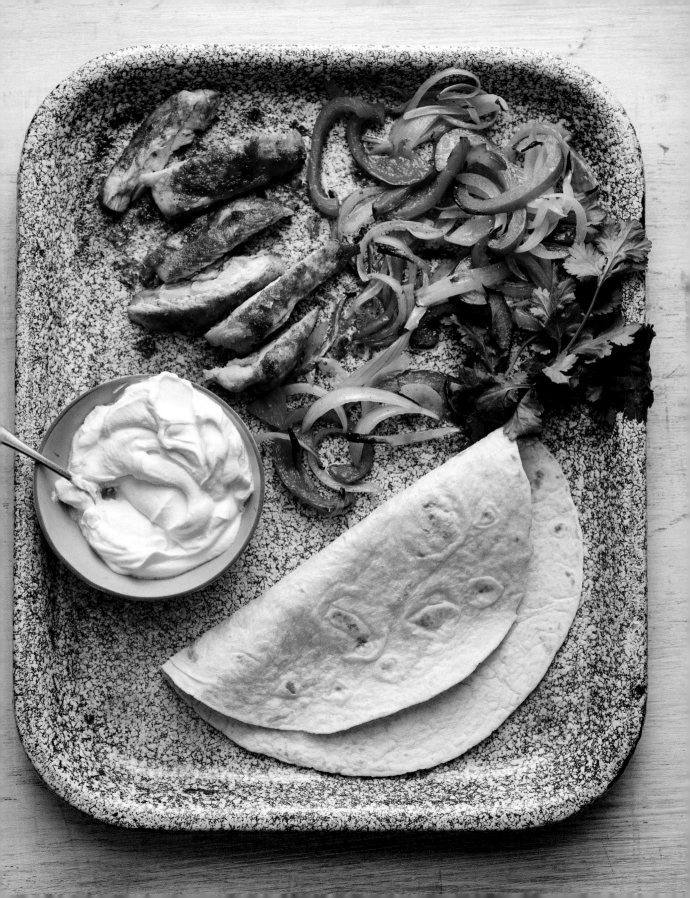

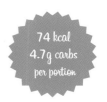

CAULIFLOWER CHOP WITH CAPER SALSA VERDE

Salsa verde is a refreshing, zingy sauce that can transform any dish into something special, and it also looks spectacular. It goes really well with the humble cauliflower; just make sure you get some colour on the veg, because that's how to get that meaty flavour into the dish. This combo is delicious, low in carbs and very low in calories.

To make 1 portion

1 slice of cauliflower, about 2cm thick

2 tbsp capers, roughly chopped plus a splash of the brine

Handful of parsley, roughly chopped

1 garlic clove, grated

Olive oil

Salt and pepper

To cook

Drizzle the cauliflower with oil and season with salt and pepper. Pan-fry over a medium heat for about 7 minutes on each side, or until cooked through and nicely coloured on the outside.

Meanwhile, combine the capers and parsley in a bowl. Add the garlic, a big glug of olive oil and a big splash of brine from the caper jar. Mix together and spoon over the cauliflower chop to serve.

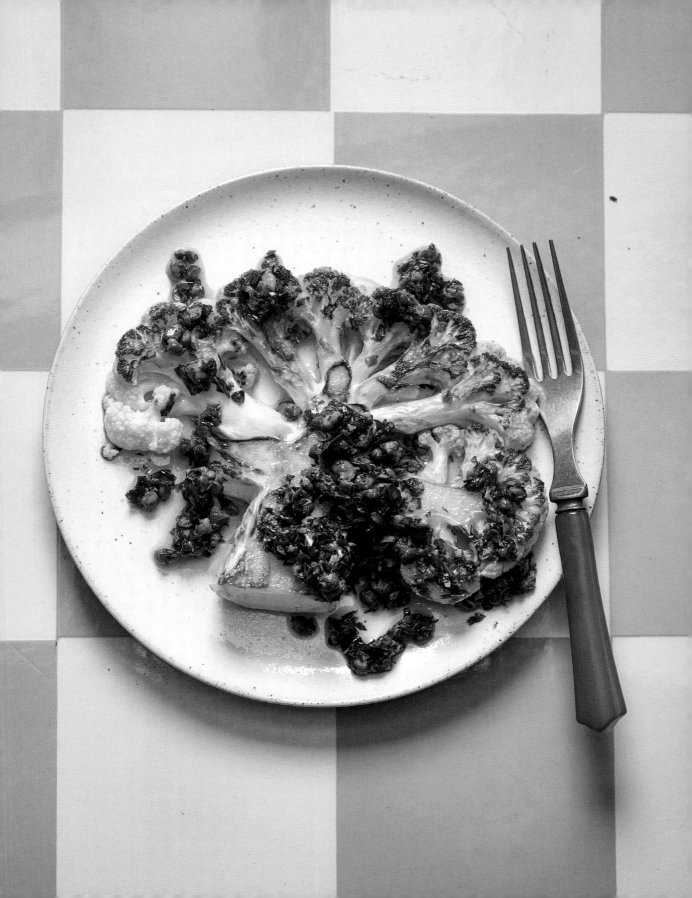

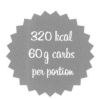

320 kcal
60g carbs
per portion

CHARRED VEG PAELLA

I experimented with cooking this dish in one pan and also cooking the rice and veg separately, and I came to the conclusion that cooking them separately means none of the flavour from the charred veg gets lost – and that's exactly how I want it.

To make 1 portion

½ onion, diced

1 garlic clove, sliced

50g paella (or risotto) rice

1 vegetable stock cube

200ml water

Pinch of saffron (optional)

½ courgette, thinly sliced lengthways

1 red pepper, seeded and sliced

½ red onion, thinly sliced

Pinch of dried oregano

Oil (any)

Salt and pepper

To cook

Pan-fry the white onion in a splash of oil over a medium heat for about 5 minutes until softened. Add the garlic and cook for a further minute. Stir in the rice and continue to cook for a few more minutes before crumbling in the stock cube and adding the water and the saffron, if using. Simmer over a low–medium heat for about 20 minutes, or until the water has been absorbed and the rice is cooked (add more water if needed, but do not stir; just let it bubble without touching it).

Meanwhile, toss the slices of courgette, red pepper and red onion in a drizzle of oil and a sprinkle of salt, pepper and oregano. Pan-fry in a griddle pan (or normal frying pan) over a high heat until cooked through and nicely charred.

Once the paella is cooked, top with the charred veg to serve.

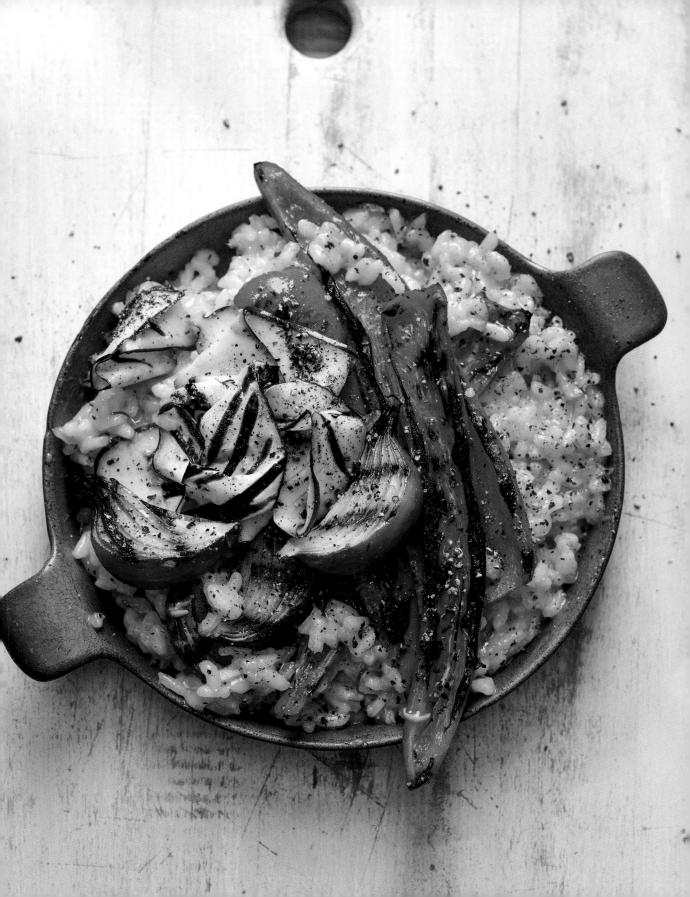

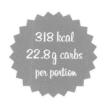

318 kcal
22.8g carbs
per portion

JAMMY ONION MOROCCAN CHICKEN

If you roast onions with chicken, they go all jammy and delicious with zero effort. So, I have used this to create the perfect Moroccan-spiced chicken with chickpeas. It all cooks at the same time, in the same dish, as if by magic.

To make 1 portion

1 large onion, cut into thin wedges

1 garlic clove, sliced

¼ tin of chickpeas (100g), drained

1 chicken leg, skin on

½ tsp smoked paprika

½ tsp ground cumin

Small handful of chopped parsley (optional)

Oil (any)

Salt and pepper

To cook

Preheat your oven to 180°C/gas mark 4.

Combine the onions, garlic and chickpeas in an ovenproof dish. Season with salt and pepper, then place the chicken on top. Drizzle with oil and sprinkle over some more salt and pepper, along with the paprika and cumin. Roast for about 30 minutes, or until the chicken is cooked through and its skin is golden brown. Garnish with parsley, if using, and serve.

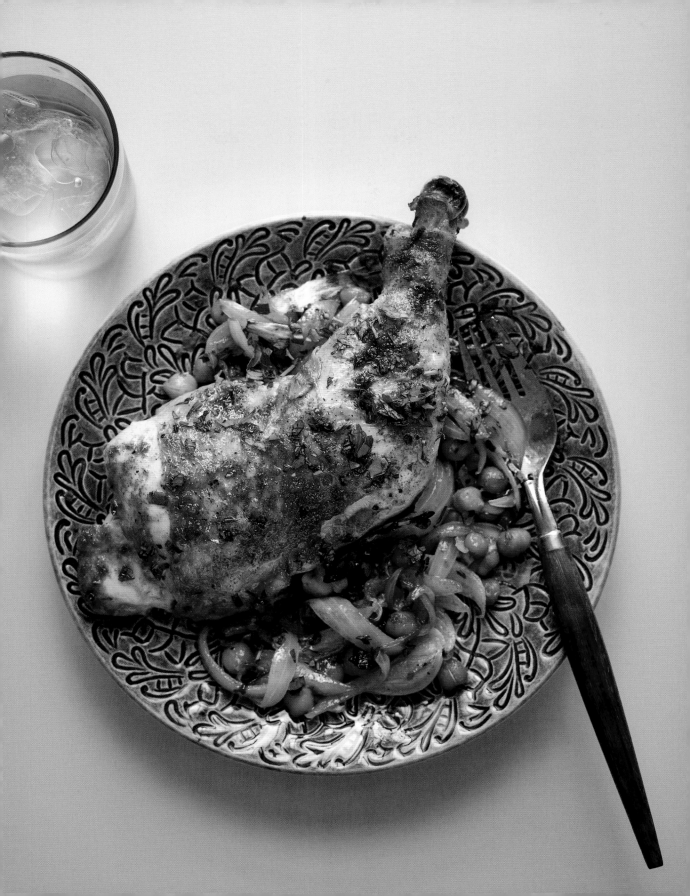

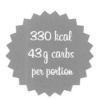

330 kcal
43g carbs
per portion

FRESH TOMATO ORZO

Sometimes you have tomatoes to use up that are past their prime – it just happens, it's part of life. This is how I deal with the problem: I make this simple orzo. It doesn't matter what kind of tomatoes you have; if you're using big tomatoes, just chop them up more.

To make 1 portion

½ onion, diced

1 garlic clove, grated

Handful of cherry tomatoes, halved

¼ mug of water

Handful of orzo

Small handful of crumbled feta

Oil (any)

Salt and pepper

To cook

Pan-fry the onion in a splash of oil over a medium heat for about 5 minutes, then add the garlic and continue to fry for a further minute. Add the tomatoes and let them break down for a few minutes in the pan. Add the water and orzo, season and simmer for about 10 minutes until the orzo is cooked, adding more water if needed. Serve with a sprinkle of feta and plenty of black pepper.

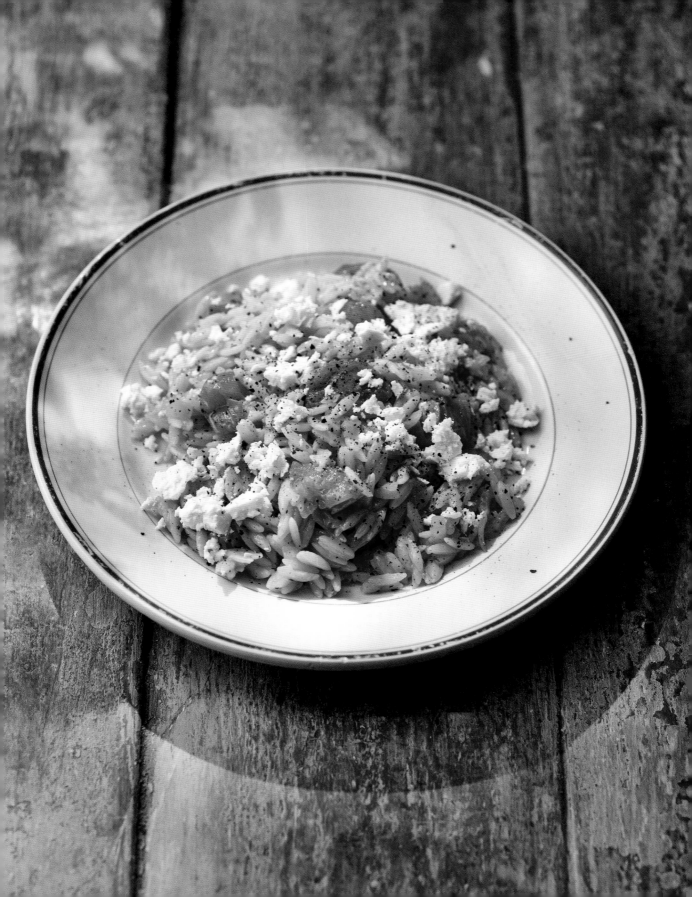

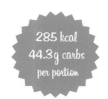
285 kcal
44.3 g carbs
per portion

INDIAN GREEN BEAN FRIED RICE

This is definitely not authentic, but it still works beautifully. If you're in a rush, you could use a packet of microwaveable rice; it's way easier. Rice is cheap, filling and low in fat, and learning a few different rice recipes will keep it interesting.

To make 1 portion

¼ mug of basmati rice

½ mug of water

¼ onion, diced

A few green beans

A small piece of fresh root ginger, grated

1 garlic clove, grated

½ tsp curry powder

1 red chilli, seeded and sliced (optional)

¼ red onion, sliced

Small handful of chopped coriander

1 tbsp natural yoghurt

Oil (any)

Salt and pepper

To cook

Put the rice and water into a saucepan with a pinch of salt and cook over a medium heat with the lid on for about 10 minutes, until all the water has been absorbed and the rice is cooked. Leave to cool.

Meanwhile, pan-fry the white onion and green beans in a splash of oil over a high heat for a few minutes until the beans are slightly charred, then add the ginger, garlic, curry powder and chilli, if using. Fry for a couple of minutes to release the flavours, then add the rice. Season, mix it all together and continue to cook for a couple of minutes. Serve topped with sliced red onion, a sprinkle of chopped coriander and a dollop of yoghurt.

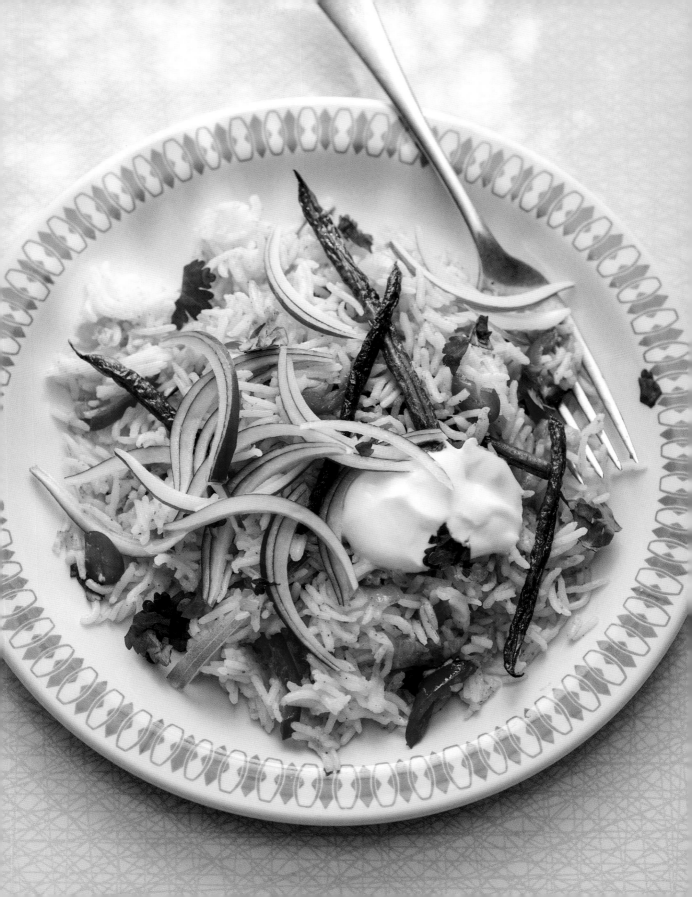

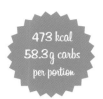

473 kcal
58.3g carbs
per portion

BLITZED CHICKPEA KORMA

The creamiest curry you can imagine, but with no cream! Instead, I've used chickpeas to create a healthy but luxurious hummus-based sauce.

To make 1 portion

¼ mug of rice

½ mug of water

¼ onion, sliced, for the sauce, plus ¼ onion, sliced, for the chicken

¼ tin of chickpeas (100g), drained

1 garlic clove, sliced

½ tsp curry powder for the sauce, plus ½ tsp for the chicken

1 skinless chicken thigh

Oil (any)

Salt and pepper

To cook

Put the rice and water into a saucepan with a pinch of salt and cook over a medium heat with the lid on for about 7 minutes, until all the water has been absorbed and the rice is cooked.

Meanwhile, pan-fry the onion for the sauce in a splash of oil for about 5 minutes until softened, then add the chickpeas, garlic and ½ teaspoon of the curry powder. Continue to fry for a few more minutes, then transfer to a blender, along with a splash of water. Blitz to create a sauce (add more water if needed) and set aside.

Rub a splash of oil, a pinch of salt and pepper and the remaining curry powder into the chicken, then pan-fry along with the remaining onion, for about 7 minutes on each side. Once cooked, slice the chicken, add it back to the pan along with the sauce. Simmer for a few minutes, then serve with the rice.

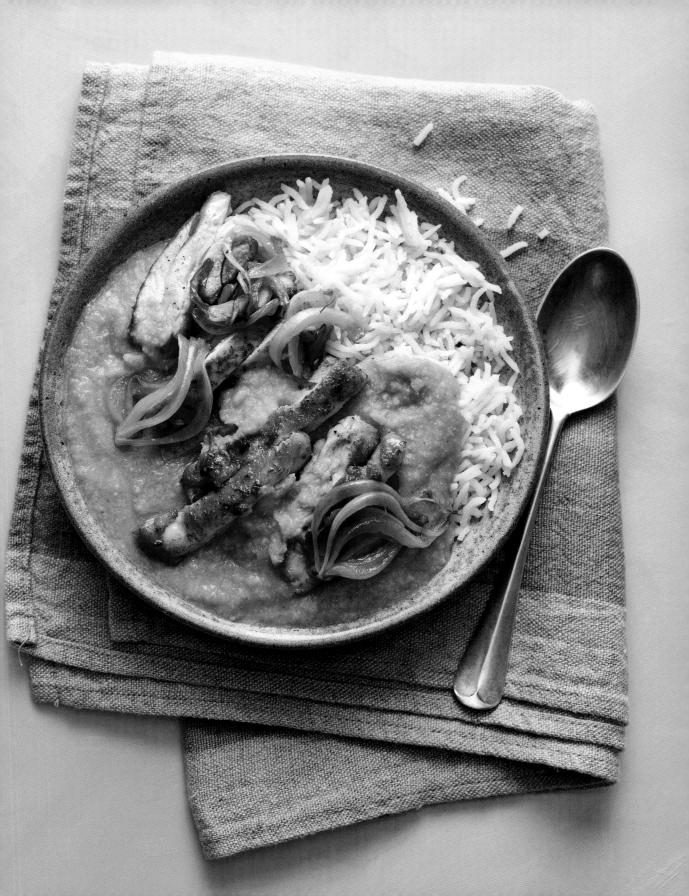

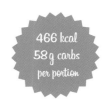

QUICK BROCCOLI & CHILLI PASTA

Cooking really doesn't get much easier than this. The pasta sauce is all veg and tastes amazing, so if you're looking for inspiration for dinner tonight, try this.

To make 1 portion

Handful of fusilli pasta

½ head of broccoli, chopped into florets

2 garlic cloves, sliced

Big pinch of dried chilli flakes

Small handful of grated Parmesan

Olive oil

Salt and pepper

To cook

Cook the pasta and broccoli in a pan of salted boiling water as per the instructions on the packet, then drain, reserving a mugful of cooking water.

Pan-fry the garlic and chilli flakes in a generous glug of olive oil over a medium heat for a couple of minutes. Add the cooked broccoli and mash with the back of a fork until the mixture looks a bit like pesto (leave some larger pieces). Season generously with salt and pepper, then add the cooked pasta, along with a splash of the cooking water, mixing everything together well.

Serve topped with a drizzle of olive oil and some grated Parmesan.

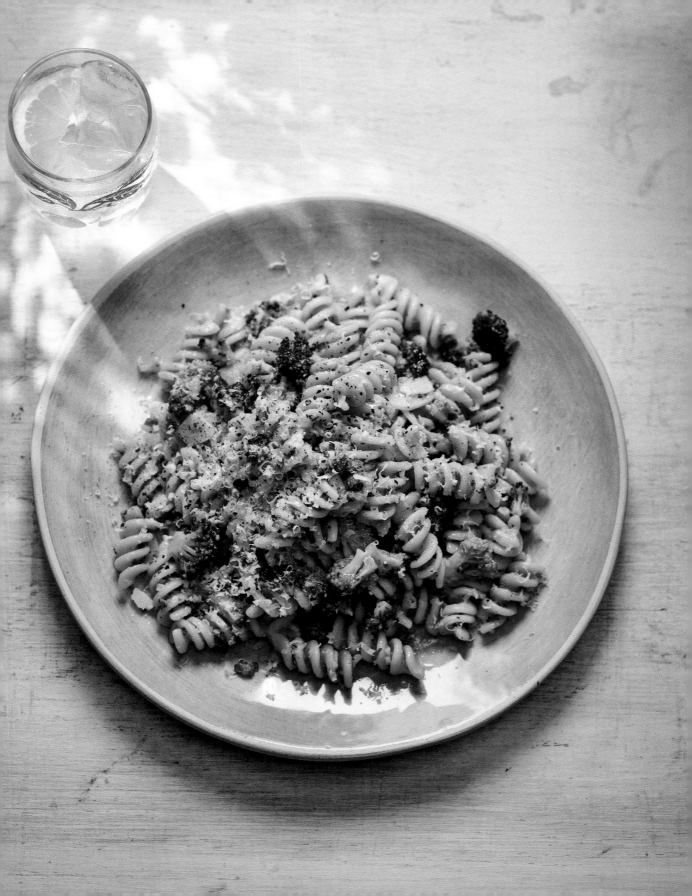

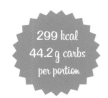

299 kcal
44.2 g carbs
per portion

KING PRAWN & CHILLI ORZO

I would describe this as an Italian-style paella. It's so easy to make. This is hearty, everyday food that is simple and quick – which is what I specialise in. To keep it cheap, make sure to use frozen prawns.

To make 1 portion

½ onion, diced

1 garlic clove, sliced

1 red chilli, seeded and sliced

200g tomato passata or ½ tin of chopped tomatoes

Handful of orzo

Handful of frozen king prawns

Handful of chopped parsley (optional)

Olive oil

Salt and pepper

To cook

Pan-fry the onion in a splash of olive oil over a medium heat for 5 minutes until softened. Add the garlic and chilli, and continue to cook for a few more minutes before adding the tomato passata or chopped tomatoes. Season well, then add the orzo and continue to simmer for about 10 minutes until the orzo is almost cooked (adding a splash of water if needed). Finally, add the prawns for the last few minutes and then serve with a sprinkle of chopped parsley, if using.

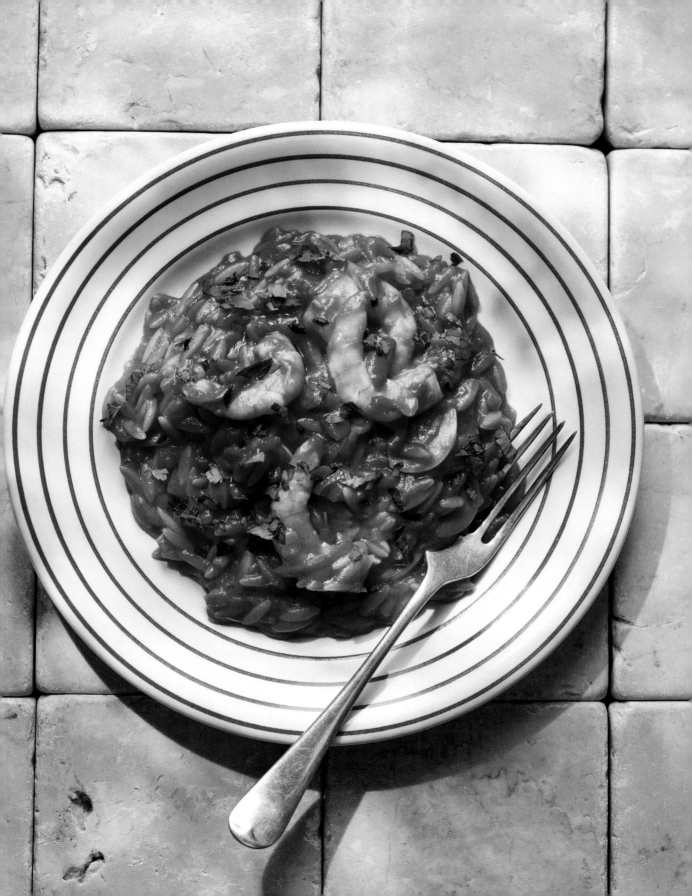

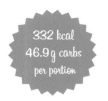

332 kcal
46.9 g carbs
per portion

CRISPY TOFU TABBOULEH

A nice twist on a classic tabbouleh, this turns it from a side dish into a lovely main course. I like to get a bit of texture into my dishes: sprinkling some breadcrumbs on top of the tofu and chucking it in the oven is by far the easiest way. Baking rather than deep-frying is a great way to reduce those unwanted extra calories.

To make I portion

Slice of tofu, about 2.5cm thick

Pinch of dried oregano

Small handful of breadcrumbs

1 garlic clove, grated

Handful of bulgur wheat

Handful of chopped parsley

1 tomato, roughly chopped

¼ red onion, diced

¼ lemon

Oil (any)

Salt and pepper

To cook

Preheat your oven to 180°C/gas mark 4 and line a baking tray.

Brush the tofu slice with oil, then season with salt, pepper and oregano. Mix the breadcrumbs with the grated garlic and some salt and pepper, then add a small splash of olive oil. Place the tofu on the lined baking tray, top with the garlic breadcrumbs and bake in the oven for about 15 minutes, or until the breadcrumbs are golden brown.

Meanwhile, cook the bulgur wheat in boiling water for 7 minutes, then drain and allow to cool a little. Mix with the parsley, tomato, red onion, a squeeze of lemon juice and a splash of oil, then season with salt and pepper.

Top the tabbouleh with the tofu and serve.

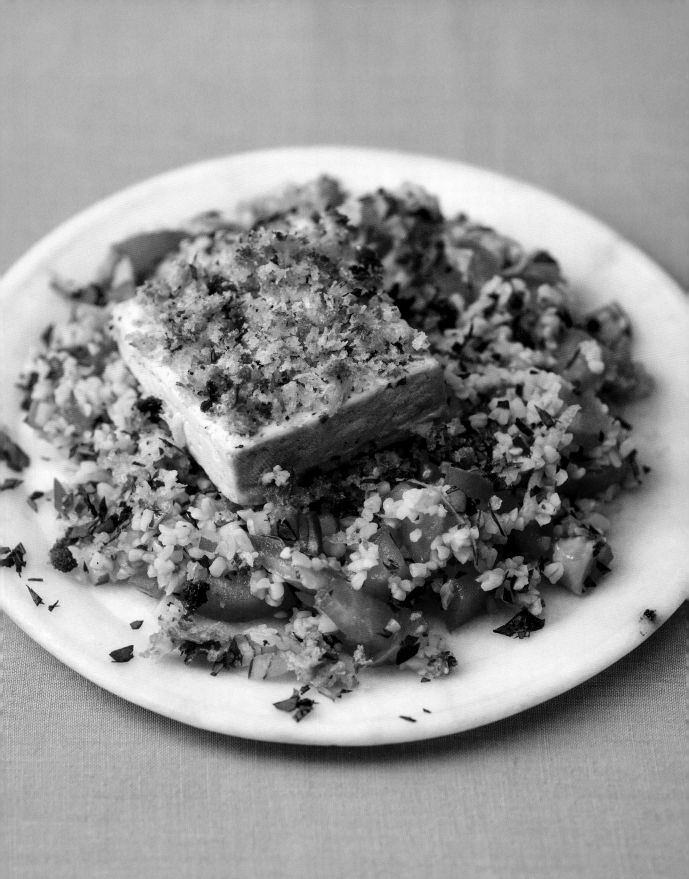

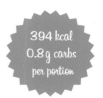

LA REINE FRITTATA

One of the easiest hot breakfasts other than toast has to be a frittata, but they make a great dinner, too. Just crack some eggs into a pan, and while they cook, rummage around in the fridge for whatever you've got left over and chuck it in. This is basically an egg-based version of a La Reine pizza! Slice the mushrooms thinly, because they won't get any direct heat, just like in a French crepe; it's a different way to enjoy mushrooms, one where they don't absorb any oil.

To make 1 portion

3 eggs

Slice of ham, cut into strips

Handful of grated Cheddar cheese

1 mushroom, thinly sliced (any variety)

Pinch of dried oregano

Oil (any)

Salt and pepper

To cook

Beat the eggs in a bowl and lightly season with salt and pepper. Pour the eggs into a small, lightly oiled frying pan over a medium heat, tilting the pan so they spread out evenly. Leave to cook for 30 seconds, or until the egg is about a quarter cooked, then throw in the ham, cheese, mushroom and oregano. Continue to cook for another minute or two, then serve once the frittata is cooked through.

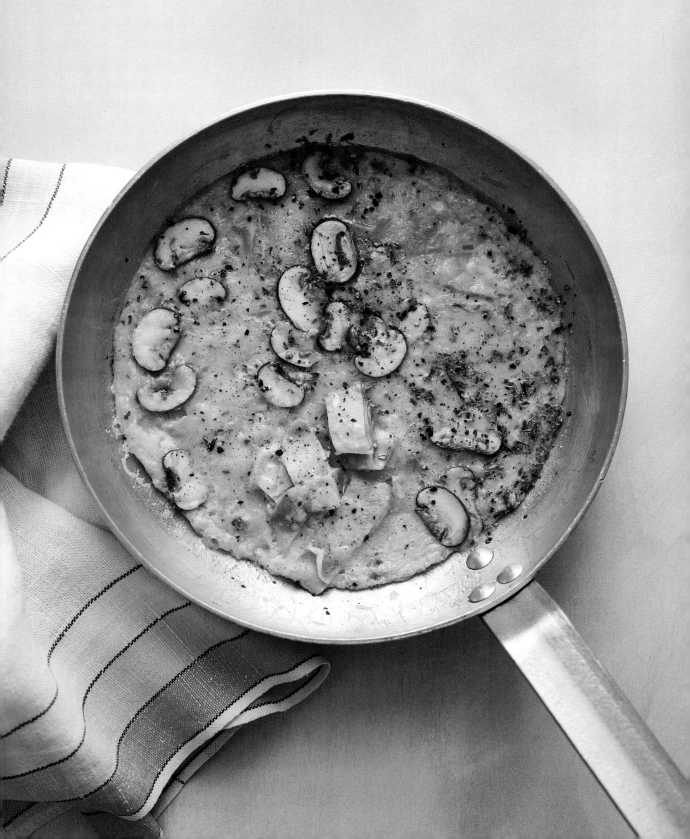

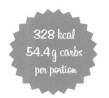

NO-CREAM STROGANOFF

I've made two clever swaps here. First, I've used milk instead of cream, which is just as tasty but with fewer calories. Second, I've used brown rice to increase the fibre and nutrient content of the dish with no extra effort.

To make 1 portion

¼ mug of brown rice

½ mug of water

A few broccoli florets

Handful of button mushrooms, sliced

½ onion, sliced

1 garlic clove, sliced

½ tsp smoked paprika

½ tsp plain flour

150ml semi-skimmed milk

Oil (any)

Salt and pepper

To cook

Put the rice and water into a saucepan with a pinch of salt and cook over a medium heat with the lid on for about 10 minutes, until all the water has been absorbed and the rice is cooked.

Meanwhile, pan-fry the broccoli and mushrooms in a splash of oil over a medium heat for about 10 minutes, then remove from the pan and set aside. Add the onion to the pan and fry in another splash of oil for about 5 minutes until softened, then add the garlic and cook for another minute or so. Season, then add the paprika and the flour. Cook for a further minute, then add the milk, little by little, stirring all the while, to create a sauce. You can add more or less milk as needed to get the perfect sauce consistency. Stir the cooked broccoli and mushrooms into the sauce and serve with the rice.

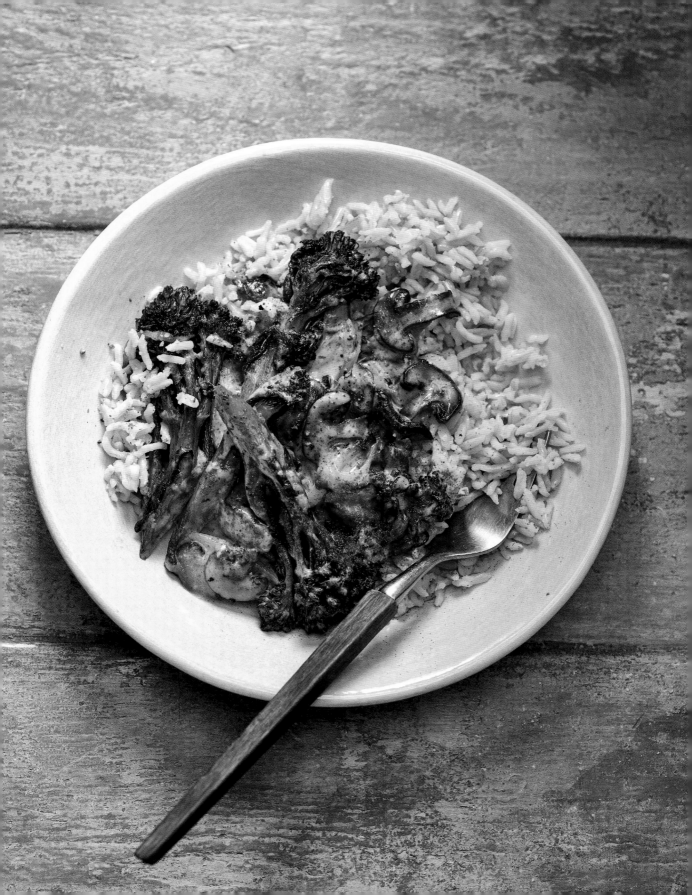

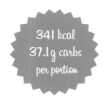

GNOCCHI ALLA NORMA

This dish can all be done in one pan, allowing the flavours to develop and limiting your washing-up. It's a nice twist on a classic, and is easy to cook even when you are busy. Aubergine is very low in calories but has a meaty texture, which makes this meal really satisfying (and also high in nutrients).

To make 1 portion

¼ aubergine, roughly chopped into chunks

1 garlic clove

Pinch of dried chilli flakes

½ tin of chopped tomatoes (200g)

Handful of gnocchi

Small handful of shaved Parmesan

Oil (any)

Salt and pepper

To cook

Pan-fry the aubergine chunks in a splash of oil over a medium heat for about 5 minutes, or until nicely coloured, then add the garlic and fry for a couple more minutes. Next, add the chilli flakes, then season and add the chopped tomatoes. Simmer for a couple of minutes, then add the gnocchi, plus a big splash of water. Simmer for a further 10 minutes, adding more water if needed. Season to taste, then serve with Parmesan.

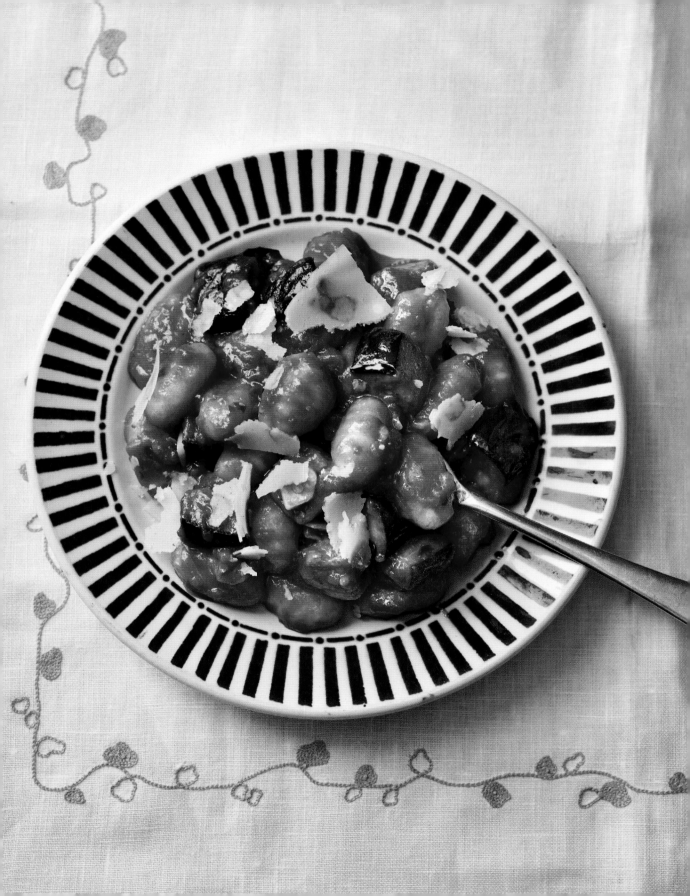

340 kcal
44.7g carbs
per portion

MISO CABBAGE CHOP

Here is a healthy alternative to meat for you to try. The key here is to get a bit of colour on the cabbage chop, which is where those ultra-savoury meaty flavours are. So don't be scared if you see a bit of charring, it's all flavour! This chop is delicious with rice – who knew you could turn two side dishes into a main meal?

To make 1 portion

¼ mug of brown rice

½ mug of water

1 tsp miso paste

½ tsp honey

Splash of soy sauce for the marinade, plus an extra splash to garnish

1 slice of white cabbage (around 2cm thick)

Small handful of chopped unsalted peanuts

Small handful of chopped chives (optional)

Salt

To cook

Preheat your oven to 180°C/gas mark 4.

Put the rice and water into a saucepan with a pinch of salt and cook over a medium heat with the lid on for about 10 minutes, until all the water has been absorbed and the rice is cooked.

Meanwhile, in a bowl, mix together the miso, honey and soy sauce to make a marinade. Place the cabbage on a baking tray, smother it with the marinade, and sprinkle over the peanuts. Roast in the oven for about 20 minutes, or until cooked through and slightly charred. Finish with a final splash of soy sauce and a sprinkle of chopped chives, if using, then serve with the rice.

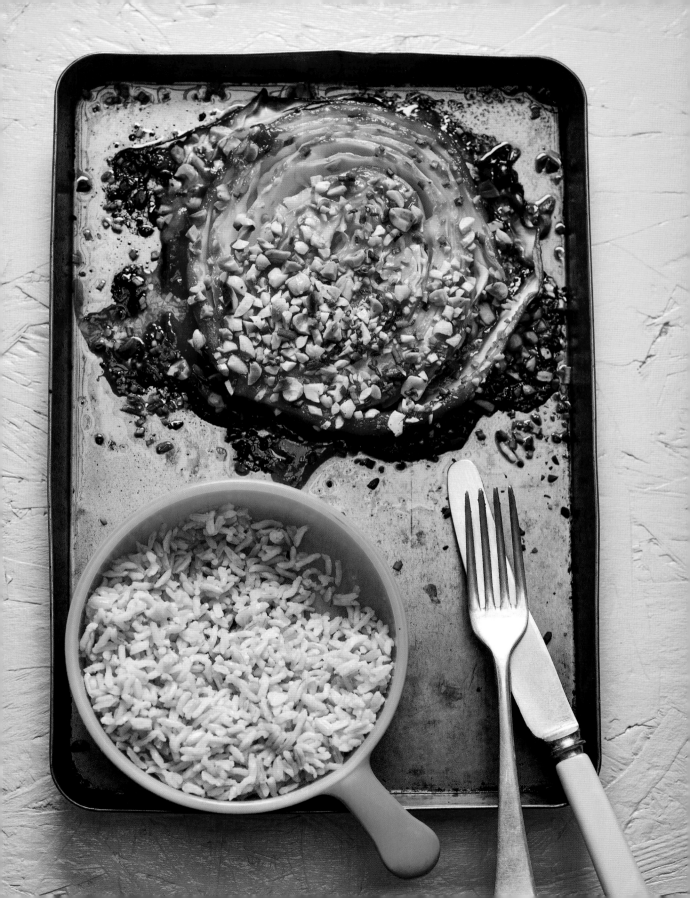

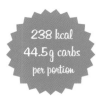

238 kcal
44.5g carbs
per portion

MUSHROOM JALFREZI

This is totally inauthentic but delicious and quick. My hack here is to use just tomato purée and curry powder. The enemy of tasty mushrooms is moisture, so a drier curry like this one works really well to magnify the flavour of the mushrooms. Plus, it satisfies that curry itch but without the calorific sauce.

To make 1 portion

¼ mug of basmati rice

½ mug of water

½ onion, sliced

Handful of sliced mushrooms (any variety)

1 tbsp tomato purée

1 garlic clove, sliced

½ tsp curry powder

Pinch of dried chilli flakes

Small handful of chopped coriander (optional)

Oil (any)

Salt and pepper

To cook

Put the rice and water into a saucepan with a pinch of salt and cook over a medium heat with the lid on for about 7 minutes, until all the water has been absorbed and the rice is cooked.

Meanwhile, pan-fry the onion and mushrooms in a splash of oil over a high heat for a few minutes, then add the tomato purée, garlic, curry powder and chilli flakes. Continue to cook for about 10 minutes, or until you see some nice caramelisation on the onions. Season to taste, then serve with the rice and garnish with a sprinkle of chopped coriander, if using.

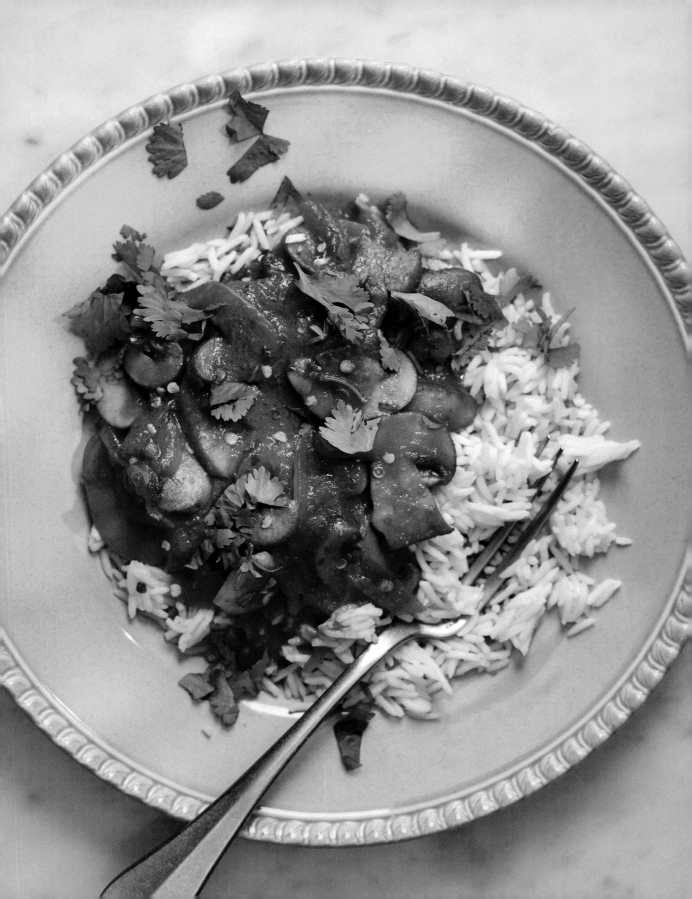

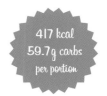

417 kcal
59.7g carbs
per portion

OVEN-BAKED SPINACH ORECCHIETTE

This dish is all done in the oven, so it's not only easy but makes hardly any mess. You could use low-fat cream cheese and skimmed milk for a lower-calorie version.

To make 1 portion

Handful of orecchiette pasta (or any small pasta)

2 tbsp cream cheese

A few pucks of frozen spinach

1 mug of semi-skimmed milk

Salt and pepper

To cook

Preheat your oven to 180°C/gas mark 4.

Grab an ovenproof dish and add the pasta, cream cheese, spinach and milk. Season well and stir it all together. Bake in the oven for about 30 minutes until the pasta is cooked. Check halfway through, giving it a stir and adding more milk, if needed.

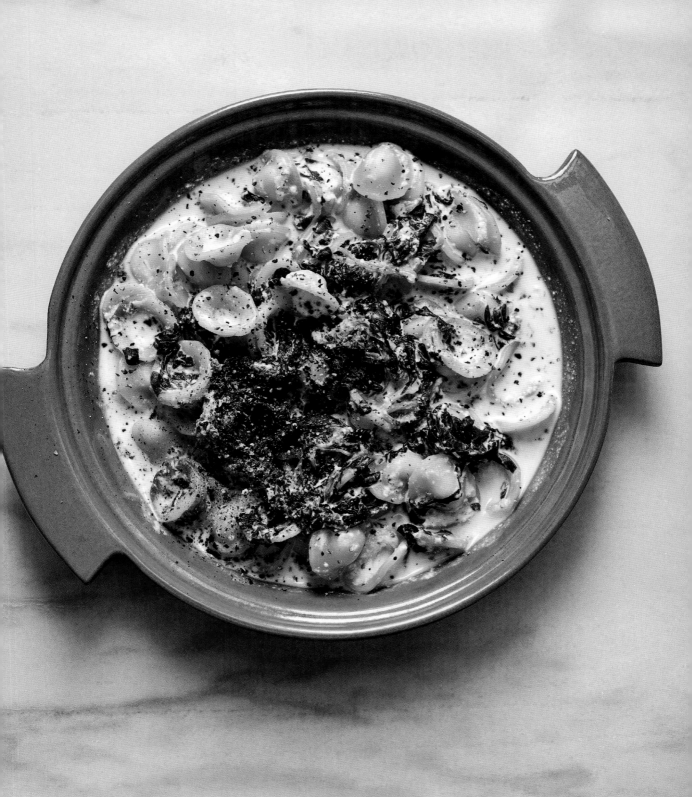

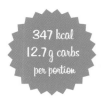

NO-CHEESE MOUSSAKA

By using a dollop of yoghurt instead of the traditional heavier béchamel-style sauce, you can transform this dish into a lower-calorie version. Roasting a whole aubergine instead of fiddling about layering up a moussaka is a useful shortcut that means it's now possible to cook this mid-week. Win win.

To make 1 portion

1 aubergine

½ red onion

Small handful of minced lamb

1 garlic clove, sliced

Pinch of ground cumin

Big dollop of natural yoghurt

Small handful of chopped parsley (optional)

Pinch of dried chilli flakes

Oil (any)

Salt and pepper

To cook

Preheat your oven to 180°C/gas mark 4.

Place the whole aubergine on a baking sheet and prick it a few times with a knife. Roast for about 30 minutes.

Meanwhile, pan-fry the onion in a splash of oil over a medium heat for a few minutes, then add the minced lamb and garlic, along with a pinch each of salt, pepper and cumin. Continue to fry for a further 8–10 minutes until the lamb is nicely coloured.

Slice the roasted aubergine lengthways down the middle, then squash it a bit with the back of a fork to open it up. Season with salt and pepper, then spoon in the lamb. Top with a dollop of yoghurt and sprinkle over some parsley, if using, and chilli flakes to garnish.

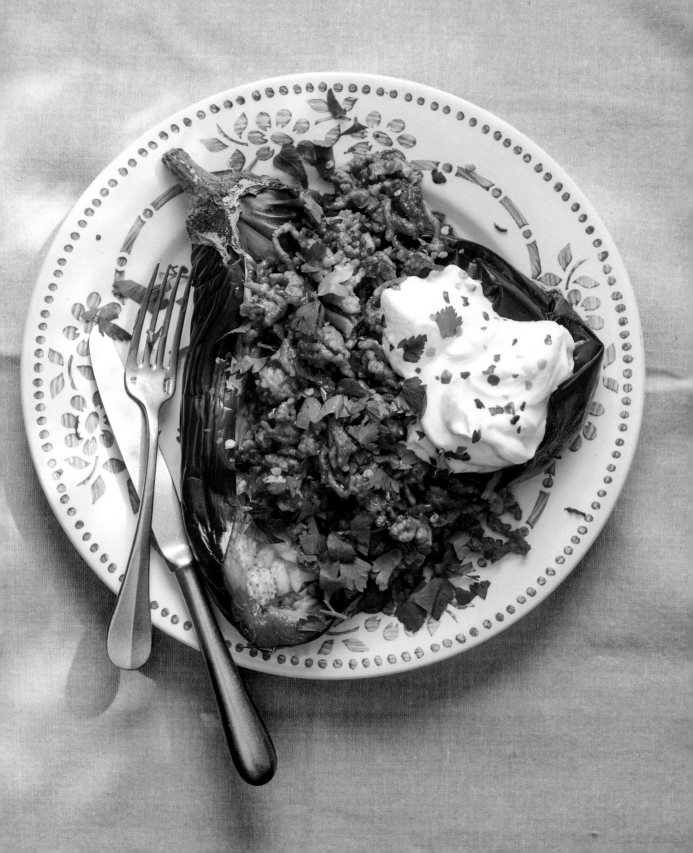

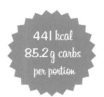

441 kcal
85.2 g carbs
per portion

ONE-PAN BURRITOS

This is such an easy meal to throw together because the filling is cooked in one pan. For a lower-carb option, you could swap the wrap for lettuce leaves.

To make 1 portion

½ onion, sliced

½ red pepper, sliced

¼ mug of rice

½ mug of water

½ tin of chopped tomatoes (200g)

½ tsp ground cumin

½ tsp smoked paprika

¼ tin of black beans (100g), drained

1 large tortilla wrap (heated, if you like)

Oil (any)

Salt and pepper

To cook

Pan-fry the onion and red pepper in a splash of oil over a medium heat for about 5 minutes before adding the rice, water, chopped tomatoes, cumin and paprika. Season and stir, then simmer for about 10 minutes until the rice is cooked, adding the black beans for the last few minutes. Spoon the mixture down the middle of the tortilla wrap, roll up and serve.

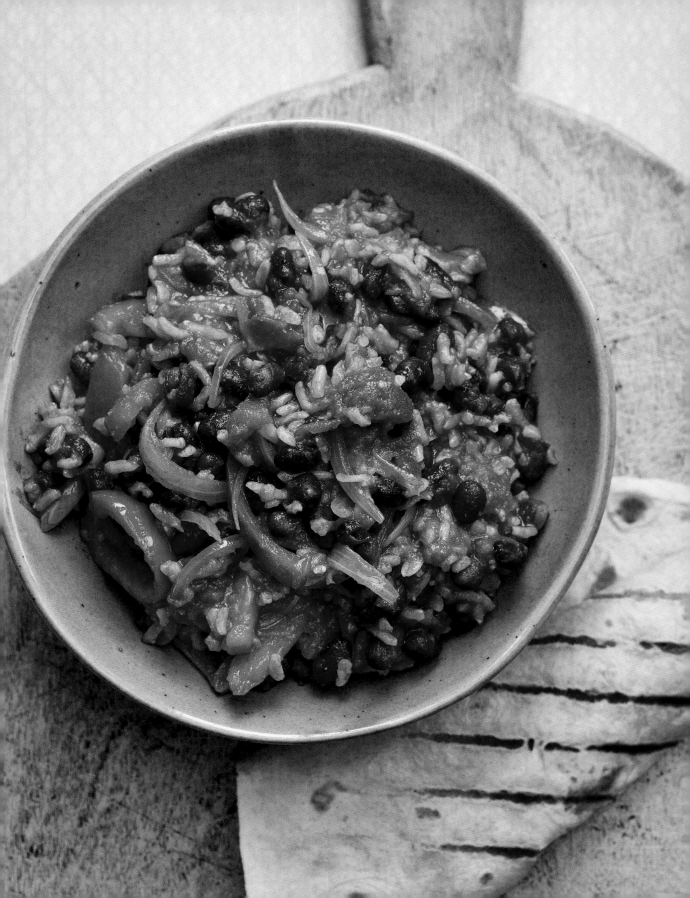

267 kcal
17.5g carbs
per portion

ONE-PAN COURGETTE PARMIGIANA

A clever little twist on the classic aubergine parmigiana. By abandoning all efforts to make it a perfectly layered masterpiece, I've created a quick and simple weeknight meal – a great example of the type of dish I like to cook. Why not try to fit a few more veg-packed meals like this into your weekly routine?

To make 1 portion

1 courgette, sliced into 3mm rounds

½ onion, sliced

1 garlic clove, sliced

½ tin of chopped tomatoes (200g)

½ tsp dried oregano

Small handful of grated Cheddar cheese

Oil (any)

Salt and pepper

To cook

Preheat the grill to high. Using a small ovenproof frying pan, fry the courgettes, along with the onion and garlic, in a splash of oil over a medium heat for about 8 minutes. Add the chopped tomatoes, then season well with salt, pepper and oregano. Simmer for about 6 minutes. Top with the Cheddar and place under the grill for a couple of minutes until the cheese is bubbling (if you don't have a frying pan with an oven-safe handle, then transfer to an ovenproof dish before putting under the grill), then serve.

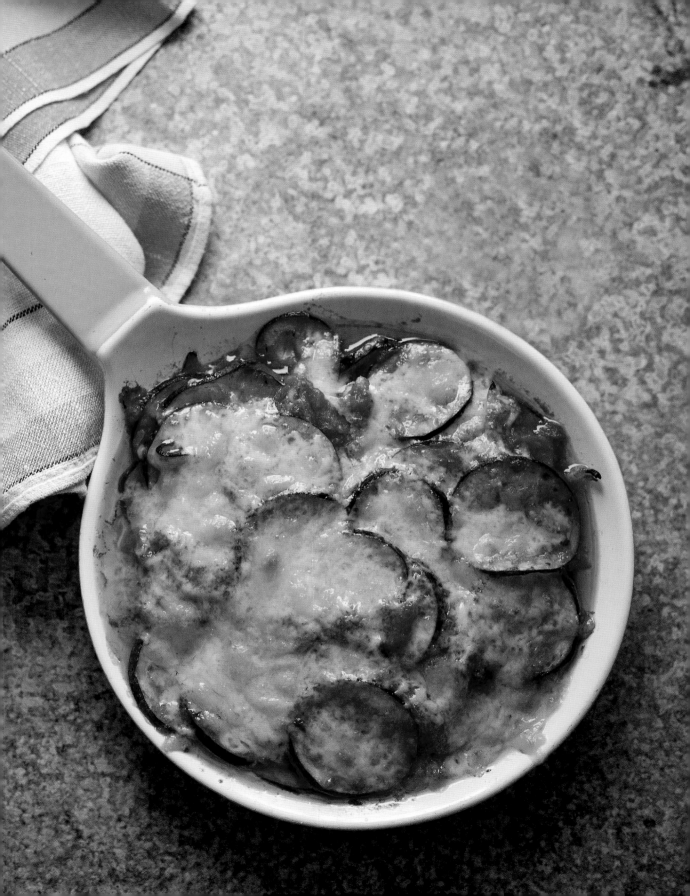

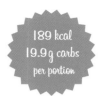

189 kcal
19.9 g carbs
per portion

OVEN AUBERGINE SCHNITZEL

The thing about breadcrumbed food is that it absorbs so much oil in the frying process. So, you have to be clever and find hacks to recreate the same crispiness but with zero oil. Baking in the oven works really well.

To make 2 schnitzels

1 aubergine, cut lengthways

Pinch of dried oregano

1 egg, beaten

Small handful of breadcrumbs

Small handful of grated Parmesan

Small handful of chopped parsley (optional)

Handful of salad leaves, to serve

Salt and pepper

To cook

Preheat your oven to 180°C/gas mark 4.

Place the aubergine on a baking sheet, skin side down. Score the aubergine flesh in a criss-cross pattern, making sure not to pierce the skin. Sprinkle with a pinch each of salt, pepper and oregano, then roast for about 15 minutes. Once softened, squash the flesh with the back of a fork to make a 'boat' and pour over the egg, then sprinkle over the breadcrumbs and Parmesan. Season once more and return to the oven for another 15 minutes, or until golden brown (keep a close eye on it, as timings will vary). Once cooked, garnish with chopped parsley, if using, and serve with salad.

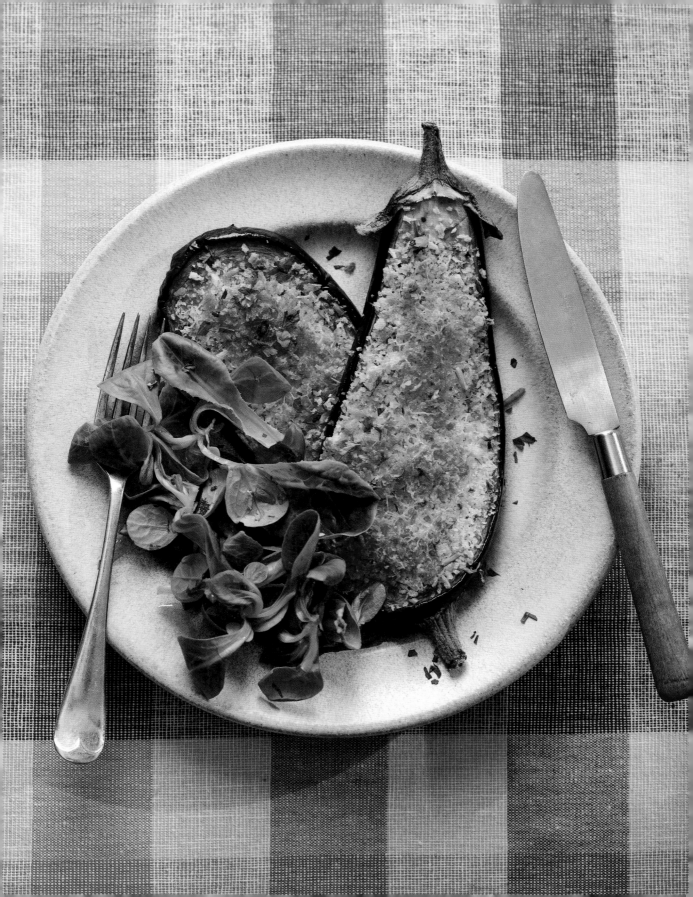

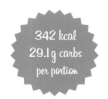

CABBAGE RIBBON & BROCCOLI ALFREDO

Ever thought of substituting pasta with cabbage? I know it sounds strange, but it works – just try this and you'll see what I'm talking about. We're not adding a whole load of cheese to the sauce here, just a little sprinkle of grated Parmesan at the end to finish the dish to perfection.

To make 1 portion

Small wedge of white cabbage, sliced into thin strips

Handful of Tenderstem broccoli pieces

1 garlic clove, sliced

Pinch of dried oregano

1 tsp plain flour

300ml any milk (including plant-based)

Small handful of grated Parmesan

Oil (any)

Salt and pepper

To cook

Season and pan-fry the cabbage and broccoli in a splash of oil over a medium heat for about 8 minutes until almost cooked, adding the garlic and oregano for the last few minutes. Next, stir in the flour. Continue to cook for another minute before adding the milk, little by little, while stirring to create a sauce. You can add more milk if the sauce is too thick. Season once more, then serve topped with a sprinkle of Parmesan.

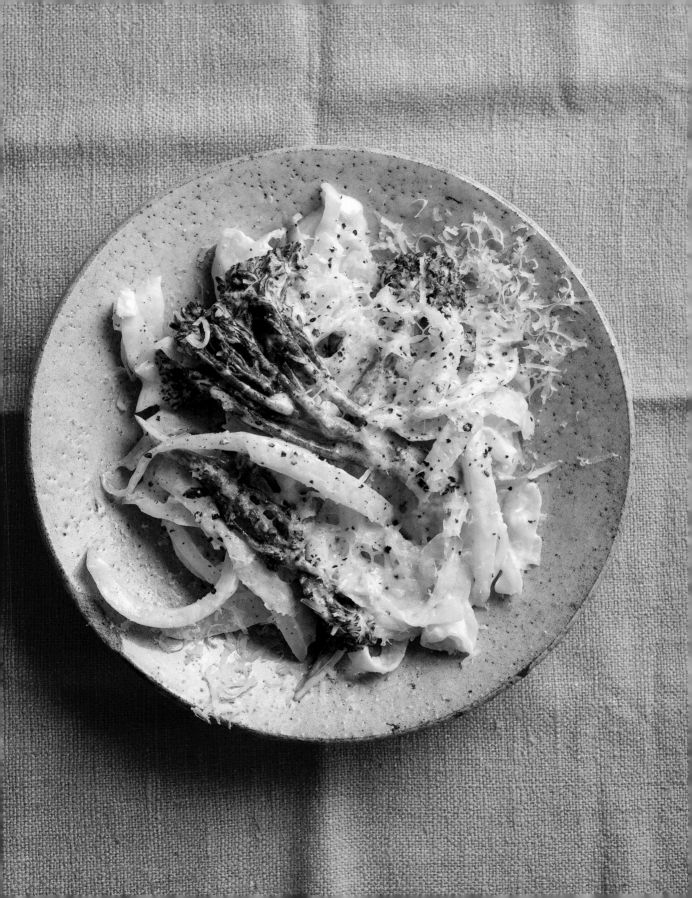

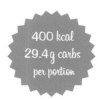

400 kcal
29.4 g carbs
per portion

SMOKED MACKEREL JOES

My take on the American sloppy Giuseppe, using crusty bread, smoked mackerel and no cheese! It's a bit like a bruschetta but more satisfying. They key here is to try and make sure the bread doesn't get too soggy, so I like to toast mine and then leave to cool before it all goes in the oven.

To make 1 portion

A few slices of crusty baguette, cut at an angle

Pinch of dried oregano

100g tomato passata

1 smoked mackerel fillet

Small handful of pitted black olives

1 garlic clove, sliced

Olive oil

Salt and pepper

To cook

Preheat your grill to high.

Rub your slices of baguette with oil, then season with salt, pepper and oregano. Toast both sides in a griddle pan or frying pan until golden brown and slightly charred. Allow to cool, then place in an ovenproof dish. Using a tablespoon, spread the passata over the bread, allowing it to drip down the sides, then flake over the mackerel and scatter over the olives and garlic. Season and drizzle with a glug of oil. Cook under the grill for about 10 minutes, keeping a close eye that it doesn't burn (timings will vary).

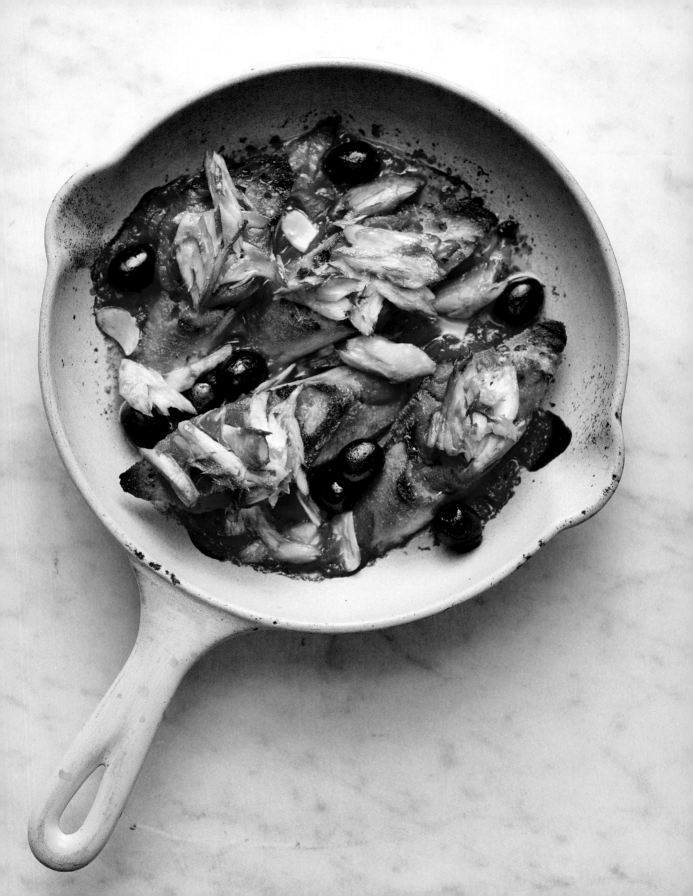

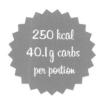

PAN-FRIED COURGETTES & ORZO

This simple dish can be knocked up in no time at all. The courgettes are the star of the show here, and by keeping them chunky, you don't need as much orzo, which lowers the carb content. Lovely hot or cold.

To make 1 portion

Handful of orzo

1 courgette, sliced

2 garlic cloves, sliced

1 thyme sprig

Olive oil

Salt and pepper

To cook

Cook the orzo in a pan of salted boiling water as per the instructions on the packet, then drain, reserving a small mugful of the cooking water.

Meanwhile, season and pan-fry the courgette slices in a splash of oil over a medium heat for about 10 minutes, adding the garlic and thyme for the last few minutes.

Add the orzo, along with a splash of the cooking water. Check the seasoning, drizzle with olive oil and serve.

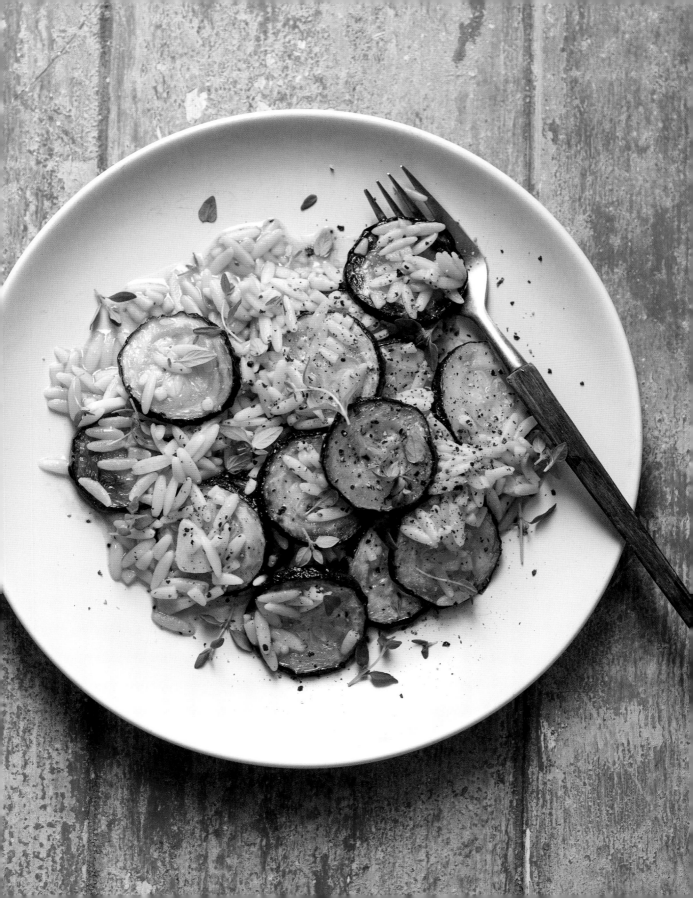

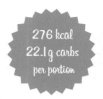

276 kcal
22.1g carbs
per portion

RED ONION & LEEK CANNELLINI BEAN STEW

Just chuck everything in a dish and let the oven do the work! The red onions are the star of the show here, rather than just being used as the base of the dish. Cannellini beans, onions and leeks are all high in fibre and nutrient-dense.

To make 1 portion

½ tin of cannellini beans (200g), plus the liquid

½ chicken stock cube (or any flavour)

Small handful of grated Cheddar cheese

½ leek, thinly sliced

1 small red onion, quartered

Oil (any)

Salt and pepper

To cook

Preheat your oven to 180°C/gas mark 4.

Tip the beans into an ovenproof dish, then crumble over the stock cube and scatter over the Cheddar and leeks. Season with salt and pepper, then place the onion quarters on top. Drizzle the onions with olive oil and season with a little more salt and pepper. Cook in the oven for about 20 minutes, then serve.

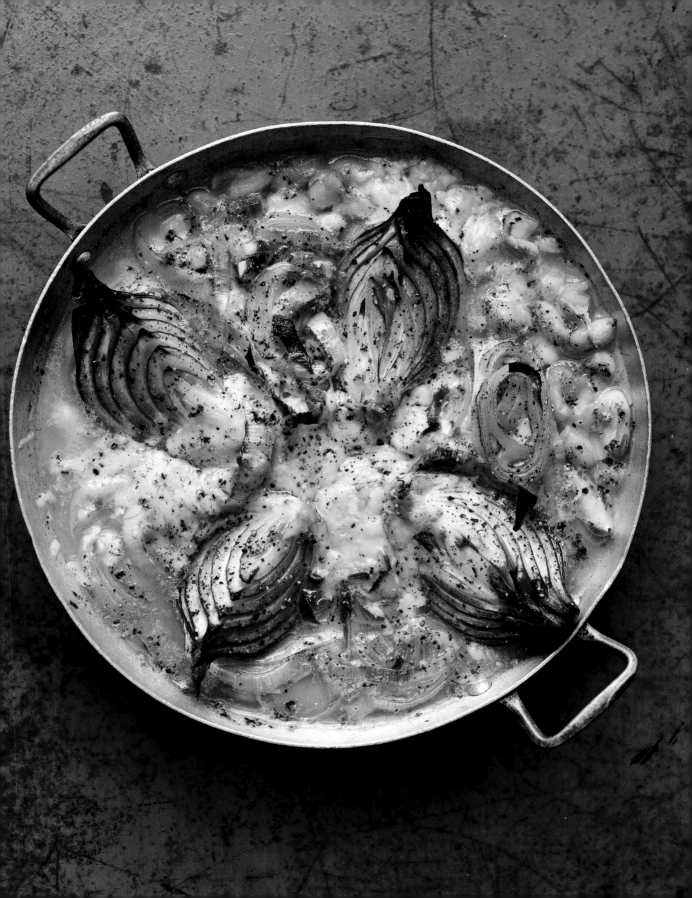

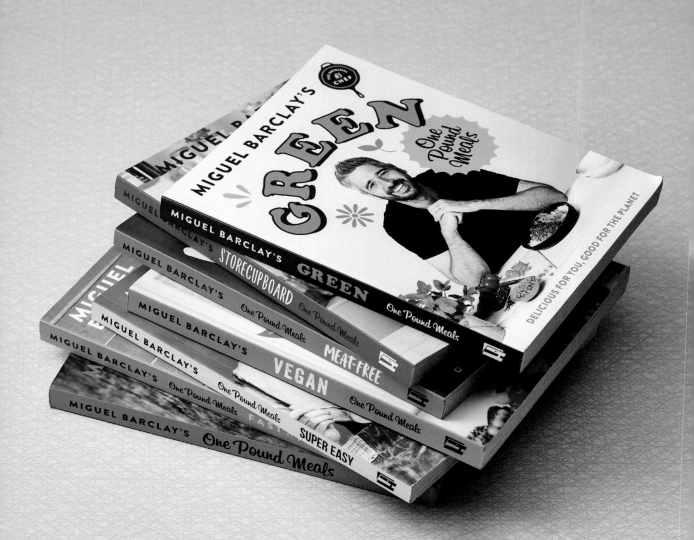

NUTRITIONAL INFO
PER PORTION

	KCAL	CARBS	FAT	SAT FAT	SUGAR	FIBRE	PROTEIN	SALT	PAGE
AUBERGINE 'BACON' BLT	260	35.7g	10.4g	1.1g	6.4g	7.5g	8.6g	0.6g	44
AUBERGINE PIZZETTE	112	5.3g	7g	4.4g	5g	3.7g	7.4g	0.3g	76
AUTUMN SALAD	403	27.9g	28.6g	9.1g	17.9g	5.9g	10.9g	0.5g	48
BACON BOLOGNESE	474	73.8g	9.5g	2.8g	20.1g	9.1g	22.5g	0.75g	102
BAKED CORN RIBS	132	12.7g	7.2g	1g	3.3g	6.9g	4.8g	0.2g	66
BAKED ZUCCHINI BALLS	379	27.3g	19.1g	7.8g	11.7g	3.8g	24.5g	0.6g	78
BEAN SPROUT NOODLES	127	15.4g	5.9g	1.2g	9.9g	6.2g	4.5g	0.2g	136
BEETROOT SALAD	279	15g	20.2g	5.7g	14.1g	4.2g	9.9g	0.4g	58
BLITZED CHICKPEA KORMA	473	58.3g	15.5g	3g	5.4g	9.3g	27.9g	0.1g	162
BOMBAY POTATO FISH CAKES	462	66.5g	8.7g	1.6g	5.3g	10.3g	31.2g	0.2g	104
BREAKFAST EGG TACOS	293	35.4g	12.7g	3.5g	2.8g	2.8g	11.5g	0.5g	24
BROKEN SPAGHETTI	473	63.7	15.3g	6.6g	10.1g	4.4g	22.8g	0.3g	118
CABBAGE RIBBON & BROCCOLI ALFREDO	342	29.1	16.2g	7.9g	19.8g	5.6g	22.5g	0.3g	190
CANNELLINI BEAN PUTTANESCA	232	7.7g	7.7g	1.2g	8.4g	10.7g	12g	0.5g	108
CASSOULET BLANCO	459	32.1g	22.9g	7.5g	8g	10.1g	29.7g	0.5g	146
CAULI BURGERS	449	52.6g	19.5g	3.2g	12.3g	5.3g	16.5g	0.5g	100
CAULIFLOWER CHOP WITH CAPER SALSA VERDE	74	4.7g	5g	0.8g	2.7g	2.1g	2.7g	0.2g	152
CAULIFLOWER GNOCCHI	239	37.8g	7.1g	1.9g	3.8g	3.9g	8.5g	0.05g	140

NUTRITIONAL INFO
PER PORTION

	KCAL	CARBS	FAT	SAT FAT	SUGAR	FIBRE	PROTEIN	SALT	PAGE
CHARRED GREEN BEAN STEW	218	32.7g	2g	0.4g	14.9g	14.2g	14.2g	0.4g	144
CHARRED VEG PAELLA	320	60g	5.8g	0.9g	15.4g	5.9g	7.5g	0.6g	154
CHICKEN & ROOT VEG HOTPOT	387	47.8g	13.4g	3g	12.3g	9.4g	20.9g	0.4g	114
CHICKEN ROMESCO	362	37.7g	14.3g	3.2g	6.5g	3.9g	21.8g	0.1g	110
CHORIZO & CHICKPEA STEW	497	54.4g	20.8g	5.5g	15.5g	15.7g	23.4g	0.8g	134
CHORIZO-STUFFED RED PEPPERS	338	35.3g	17.7g	5.4g	8.6g	2.8g	11.3g	0.5g	56
COCONUT CURRY	469	24.6g	38.9g	30g	15.1g	6g	6.8g	0.03g	106
COURGETTE LASAGNE	337	27.8g	16.6g	7.3g	25.7g	7.1g	18.1g	0.4g	120
CREAMY PUMPKIN SOUP WITH SAGE CROUTONS	192	30.2g	6.3g	1.1g	10.7g	5.7g	6.1g	0.4g	70
CRISPY CHICKPEA SHAKSHUKA	226	17g	11.4g	2.1g	6.4g	4.8g	12.7	0.4g	38
CRISPY MUSHROOM PANCAKES	199	28g	6.7g	0.8g	11.3g	3.5g	5.1g	0.5g	72
CRISPY TOFU TABBOULEH	332	46.9g	10.6g	1.5g	6.1g	5.3g	15.4g	0.1g	168
EGG KRAPOW	366	44.2g	14.1g	3.3g	1.5g	2.7g	18.2g	0.2g	96
FILO PASTRY BROCCOLI TART	500	49.7	26.4g	7.3g	7g	3.4g	14.8g	1g	84
FLATTENED CHICKEN WITH CAPER JUS	151	0.3g	5.8g	1g	0g	0.3g	24.2g	0.3g	116
FRESH TOMATO ORZO	330	43g	11.8	5g	7.7g	3.7g	12.7g	0.3g	158
FROZEN PRAWN PHO	255	39.7g	5.2g	0.9g	1.1g	1.8g	11.9g	0.6g	94
GNOCCHI ALLA NORMA	341	37.1g	14.2g	6.7g	9.7g	4.5g	16.6g	0.4g	174

NUTRITIONAL INFO
PER PORTION

	KCAL	CARBS	FAT	SAT FAT	SUGAR	FIBRE	PROTEIN	SALT	PAGE
GREEK POTATO SALAD	233	21.5g	12.7g	5.1g	4g	3.5g	7.5g	0.5g	62
HALLOUMI CHOPPED SALAD	372	11.7g	26.4g	8.7g	9.2g	5.4g	21.4g	0.7g	52
HAM & MUSTARD REMOULADE TARTE	329	49.9g	8g	2.2g	8.6g	3.2g	12.6g	0.4g	50
HONEY NUT & CRANBERRY GRANOLA	354	57.6	11.3g	1.1g	28.9g	6.1g	7.9g	0.2g	28
INDIAN GREEN BEAN FRIED RICE	285	44.3g	9.7g	3.8g	7.6g	3.6g	7.8g	0.04g	160
JAMMY ONION MOROCCAN CHICKEN	318	22.8g	11.7	2.1g	9.8g	6.4g	28.4g	0.1g	156
KING PRAWN & CHILLI ORZO	299	44.2g	5.9g	0.9g	8.5g	3.9g	16.9g	0.1g	166
LA REINE FRITTATA	394	0.8g	29.4g	11.2g	0.4g	0.5g	31.3g	0.6g	170
LEMON BROCCOLI COUSCOUS BOWL	422	34.1g	25.7g	5.9g	3.1g	4g	15.1g	0.3g	88
LENTIL CHILLI BOWL	470	75.8g	9.7g	2.7g	14.1g	15.6g	23.4g	0.5g	126
MEXICAN FAUX-PASTRY WRAPS	483	67.1g	12.4g	2.4g	13.1g	17.2g	25.1g	0.4g	92
MISO CABBAGE CHOP	340	44.7g	14.5g	2.4g	9.1g	g	10g	0.6g	176
MUSHROOM JALFREZI	238	44.5g	5.6g	0.9g	7.7g	3.6g	5.8g	0.01g	178
NO-BOIL PASTA BAKE	500	67.3g	14.3g	8.8g	13.8g	5.9g	24.1g	0.3g	122
NO-CHEESE MOUSSAKA	347	12.7g	25.3g	11.1g	9.8g	7g	18.7g	0.1g	182
NO-CHEESE RISOTTO	278	43.4g	1.4g	0.3g	6.9g	3.5g	14.2g	0.5g	124
NO-CREAM STROGANOFF	328	54.4g	8.3g	2.5g	13.3g	5.8g	12.9g	0.07g	172
ONE-PAN BURRITOS	441	85.2g	4.8g	1.8g	17g	11.4g	15.8g	0.48g	184

NUTRITIONAL INFO
PER PORTION

	KCAL	CARBS	FAT	SAT FAT	SUGAR	FIBRE	PROTEIN	SALT	PAGE
ONE-PAN COURGETTE PARMIGIANA	267	17.5g	15.9g	7.3g	15.6g	4.9g	13.2g	0.3g	186
OVEN AUBERGINE SCHNITZEL	189	19.9g	7.1g	2.5g	3.9g	4.8g	12.3g	0.2g	188
OVEN BHAJIS	208	37.2g	1.6g	0.2g	14.3g	5.3g	10.6g	0.05g	60
OVEN-BAKED SPINACH ORECCHIETTE	417	59.7g	10.8g	6.4g	9.3g	3.1g	18.9g	0.2g	180
OVEN-ROASTED TOMATO SOUP	109	12.8g	5.5g	0.8g	10.2g	4.2g	3g	0.2g	80
OVERNIGHT OATS	420	65.2g	14.3g	3.3g	31.4g	6.4g	12g	0.2g	36
PAN-FRIED COURGETTES & ORZO	250	40.1g	5.7g	0.9g	5.1g	2.5g	9.1g	0.02g	194
PASTA ALLA SORRENTINA	408	57.2g	2.4g	5.2g	5g	3.3g	15.8g	0.1g	142
PEANUT BUTTER BREAKFAST BARS (PER BAR)	98	13.3g	3.9g	0.6g	6g	1.2g	0.3g	0.2g	40
POACHED CHICKEN NOODLE SOUP	359	51.9g	3.2g	0.6g	8.2g	5.3g	30.5g	0.6g	86
POACHED EGG RAMEN	263	30.9g	10g	2g	1.4g	0.8g	12.1g	0.5g	46
POLENTA & TINNED CHERRY TOMATOES	317	28.7g	16.5g	7.4g	13.5g	5.6g	13.7g	1g	138
QUICK BROCCOLI & CHILLI PASTA	466	58g	15.2g	6.8g	3.9g	5.9g	24.3g	0.2g	164
RED ONION & LEEK CANNELLINI BEAN STEW	276	22.1g	12.5g	5.3g	6.1g	10.4g	15.3g	0.2g	196
ROCKET PESTO LASAGNE SHEETS	327	30.5g	19g	1.7g	1.8g	2.1g	8.4g	0.2g	128
SAVOURY BREAKFAST YOGHURT	487	35.5g	28.3g	14.3g	11.1g	2.4g	21.6g	0.5g	30
SAVOY CABBAGE EGG	258	3.3g	18.2g	4.5g	2.5g	1.9g	20.3g	0.7g	64

NUTRITIONAL INFO
PER PORTION

	KCAL	CARBS	FAT	SAT FAT	SUGAR	FIBRE	PROTEIN	SALT	PAGE
SMASHED PEA, AVOCADO & FETA	318	35.3g	14.4g	6g	4.4g	7.2g	13.9g	0.6g	34
SMOKED MACKEREL JOES	400	29.4g	23.2g	4.5g	4.3g	3g	19.4g	0.87g	192
SMOKED SALMON ROSTI HACK	334	41.9g	12.5g	4g	2.4g	4.7g	14.7g	0.5g	32
SMOKY BEANS ON TOAST	361	44.7g	11.7g	2.5g	8.9g	10.2g	19.3g	0.5g	22
SPICED CARROT & LENTIL SOUP	233	32.8g	8g	2.4g	15.6g	12.3g	9.5g	0.05g	54
STICKY BLACK PEPPER NOODLES	210	32.5g	5.6g	0.8g	3g	2.6g	7.4g	0.2g	130
SUN-DRIED TOMATO & ASPARAGUS ORZO	320	44.8g	10.2g	3.2g	8.7g	6.7g	11g	0.5g	132
SUN-DRIED TOMATO PESTO GNOCCHI	306	28.4g	18.6g	1.7g	1.1g	2.3g	6g	0.2g	112
TEXAN SALSA SALAD	333	42.2g	11.8g	1.4g	9.5g	14.6g	11.4g	0.1g	82
THE RACHEL SALAD	390	36.8g	20.9g	6.1g	4.7g	6g	14.6g	0.3g	74
TOFU ALMONDINE	266	12.1g	17.9g	2.1g	1.9g	3.7g	14.4g	0.06g	68
TOFU RENDANG	408	49.3g	14.6g	2.7g	12.6g	4.9g	22g	0.2g	148
TOMATO & BACON BREAKFAST OMELETTE	361	6.1g	22.8g	6.1g	4.5g	2.7g	33.1g	0.8g	26
TRAY-BAKE FAJITAS	425	44.6g	18.4g	5.9g	9.7g	4.9g	22.1g	0.5g	150
YOGHURT CAESAR SALAD	342	33.2g	16.9g	7.8g	11.7g	3.8g	24.5g	0.6g	90

INDEX

The author worked on the recipes with Sophie Elletson DipNT CNM mNNA,
a Registered Nutritional Therapist and lead nutritionist at FUTURE WOMAN.

First published in 2023 by Headline Home
an imprint of Headline Publishing Group

1

Cataloguing in Publication Data is available from the British Library

ISBN 978 1035 40395 0
eISBN 978 1035 40396 7

Commissioning Editor: Lindsey Evans   Design: Superfantastic
Senior Editor: Kate Miles   Photography: Dan Jones
Copy Editor: Sophie Elletson   Photography Assistant: Rosie Alsop
Page Make-up: EM&EN   Food Styling: Natalie Thomson
Proofreaders: Tara O'Sullivan and Ilona Jasiewicz   Food Styling Assistant: Sophie Edwards
Indexer: Ruth Ellis   Prop Styling: Christina Mackenzie

Colour reproduction by ALTA London
Printed and bound in Italy by L.E.G.O. S.p.A.

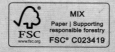

Headline's policy is to use papers that are natural, renewable and recyclable products
and made from wood grown in sustainable forests. The logging and manufacturing processes
are expected to conform to the environmental regulations of the country of origin.

HEADLINE PUBLISHING GROUP
An Hachette UK Company
Carmelite House
50 Victoria Embankment
London EC4Y 0DZ

www.headline.co.uk
www.hachette.co.uk